"Dr. Galanter uses his experience as a leading specialist in the field to explore the world's most prolific program helping millions struggling with the disease of addiction. *What is Alcoholics Anonymous?* should be on the bookshelves of anyone who has been touched by or cares about this illness."
—Christopher Kennedy Lawford, NY Times bestselling author and recovery activist

"A true masterpiece! It captures the essence of hope and how paramount it is for recovering people to carry the message to those still suffering."
—John Shinholser, President, McShin Recovery Resource Foundation

"In this book, Dr. Marc Galanter, a distinguished pioneer in addiction studies and treatment, benefits the reader with his experience and knowledge spanning decades in explaining how AA works and helps those who attend the program."
—Edward J. Khantzian, MD, Professor of Psychiatry, Harvard Medical School

"*What is AA?* escapes the pro-AA and anti-AA polemics of recent years and instead conveys the author's knowledge and experience in a most engaging style. It will find highly appreciative audiences among individuals seeking escape from alcohol-related problems, affected family members, and a wide range of helping professionals, particularly those working on the frontlines of addiction treatment."
—William L. White, MA, Author, *Slaying the Dragon: The History of Addiction Treatment in America*

"The road to recovery is sometimes a long and winding one. Dr. Galanter's book explains how to navigate the bumps and distractions. The best explanation of Alcoholics Anonymous on the market: honest and revealing."
—Pat O'Brien, NY Times bestselling author

"Dr. Galanter does an excellent job of demystifying AA and sheds much-needed light on the workings of the AA fellowship. Perhaps it will surprise some that 12-step recovery *is* an evidence-based treatment that can be highly effective and certainly measures up favorably against other treatment processes."
—Dr. Drew Pinsky, Host of TV talk show "Dr. Drew On Call," and Assistant Clinical Professor of Psychiatry at the Keck School of Medicine of USC

"This book harnesses the firm science of addiction and recovery and enhances it with the humanness of deeply personal anecdotes from those who have overcome their seemingly hopeless condition. Most of all, it gives the reader what is essential to anyone taking that first step on the journey to recovery: hope."
—William C. Moyers, Vice President, Hazelden Betty Ford Foundation

"Dr. Galanter, an addiction psychiatrist, master clinician, scholar, and educator, has provided an accessible overview of AA. It will be useful for a broad range of readers who wish to know more about this ubiquitous but often misunderstood peer-led recovery program. It should be useful in demystifying AA and diminishing barriers for individuals with alcohol problems who are considering using this program."
—Shelly Greenfield MD, MPH, Professor of Psychiatry, Harvard Medical School

"This book is the most authoritative work on AA's role in addiction recovery yet written. It is highly engaging, and meets the need for information that is objective and unbiased, available in no other source. It combines compelling examples of recovery with related research, including neuroscience, to back up its conclusions."
—Gregory Bunt, MD, President, International Society of Addiction Medicine

What is Alcoholics Anonymous?

WHAT IS ALCOHOLICS ANONYMOUS?

A Path from Addiction to Recovery

Marc Galanter, MD

Professor of Psychiatry and Director,
Division of Alcoholism and Drug Abuse
NYU School of Medicine

OXFORD
UNIVERSITY PRESS

Oxford University Press is a department of the University of Oxford. It furthers
the University's objective of excellence in research, scholarship, and education
by publishing worldwide. Oxford is a registered trade mark of Oxford University
Press in the UK and certain other countries.

Published in the United States of America by Oxford University Press
198 Madison Avenue, New York, NY 10016, United States of America.

Library of Congress Cataloging-in-Publication Data
Names: Galanter, Marc, author.
Title: What is Alcoholics Anonymous? : a path from addiction to recovery / Marc Galanter.
Description: Oxford ; New York : Oxford University Press, [2016] |
Includes bibliographical references.
Identifiers: LCCN 2015040579 | ISBN 9780190276560 (alk. paper)
Subjects: | MESH: Alcoholics Anonymous. |
Alcoholism—rehabilitation—Personal Narratives. | Self-Help Groups—Personal Narratives.
Classification: LCC RC565 | NLM WM 274 | DDC 616.86/106—dc23
LC record available at http://lccn.loc.gov/2015040579

CONTENTS

PREFACE

This book is the product of a diverse set of efforts, each of which played a role in my trying to answer the question posed by its title. In the late 1970s, shortly after my psychiatric training and a stint at the U.S. National Institute of Mental Health, I received a Career Teacher grant from the federal government to develop medical school training and research in the nascent field of addiction medicine. It was highly influential in the course of my career and that of other of the awardees. At the time, there was little to offer alcoholics for a stabilized recovery free of their addiction other than going to AA. It seemed important to gain an understanding of how this fellowship achieved this for many people. This federal funding was instrumental in developing initiatives that came to be central in the development of addiction medicine as an academic discipline.

I must express appreciation for the many members of Alcoholics Anonymous (AA) and Narcotics Anonymous (NA) who volunteered their time for our studies, focus groups, and interviews to shed light on their encounters with the fellowship. Their anonymity has been preserved by changing both details of their stories as needed, and their names. This personal information is balanced by findings from committed and dispassionate researchers who have undertaken studies on the nature and relative effectiveness of Twelve Step experiences. Without their findings, I would have a limited context in which to do this work.

This effort also ensues from clinical care in which I have been involved in the domain of addiction over almost a half century. Twelve Step groups are still a bulwark for many, particularly those most severely bound to alcohol and other drug addictions. So the need to understand how the fellowship achieves its effect persists, and the opportunity to approach this task has been enhanced by what we have learned over those decades. My patients have taught me much of what I know about addiction and recovery, while we have worked together to help them free themselves from the bonds of their dependencies on alcohol and other drugs. The help I have been able to afford them has been the greatest reward of my work.

Key research collaborators of mine, Drs. Helen Dermatis, Stephen Post, and Zoran Josipovich in particular, as well as my addiction psychiatry fellows, made our studies at New York University (NYU) possible. Each contributed expertise and talent particular to his or her respective discipline. Over these years, many smart and earnest research assistants have worked with us on our projects, have contributed materially to them, and have moved on to successful careers. Jim Levine, my literary agent was kind enough to represent me for this and a previous, related book. Bill Ciccaroni and Jane Nickels of AA and NA were invaluable as liaisons to the fellowships. Two assistants of mine here at NYU, Kristin Frillman and Jacqueline Howard labored with competence and intelligence as I went through endless revisions of this and other manuscripts.

The American Society of Addiction Medicine, the American Academy of Addiction Psychiatry, and the American Psychiatric Association were open to serving as vehicles for presenting the research as cited here, and Drs. Richard Ries and Penny Ziegler worked together with me in carrying this work forward in those associations.

Our research at New York University was supported by the National Institute on Drug Abuse, the Scaife Family Foundation, the Robert Wood Johnson Foundation, The Commonwealth Fund, The Badgeley Charitable Trust, and most importantly, for our most recent work, The John Templeton Foundation.

The NYU School of Medicine, dedicated to advancing treatment, research, and education, on the front lines of the battle against the many diseases people face, has been most hospitable for this work. Its Department of Psychiatry and affiliate Bellevue Hospital have been invaluable settings and resources for what we have done in this domain.

INTRODUCTION

What really goes on in AA? How can it help a person with addiction?

This book is written to meet the need for clear answers to these questions. Books published by Alcoholics Anonymous offer a potential member a way to join and get involved, but surprisingly, there is no book that looks at this fellowship from an expert and independent position and objectively spells out the answers to these questions. And answers are needed for addicted people thinking of going to AA, for their concerned family and friends, and even for professionals in the addiction field. The decision to turn to AA is too important for relying on all the conflicting voices found on the Internet or in advocacy articles, for or against it. What is needed is a way to understand AA by putting the diverse experiences of people who encounter it into the context of what the research on it can tell us.

Here is an example of the difficulty of getting an understanding of this program. Consider the words of one member:

> I couldn't tell you how it works. It just works. You couldn't have told me that
> I would never use alcohol or a drug for these last thirteen years. I would have
> bet anything against it. So to me it's a true miracle that I am able to stay sober.

This was told to me by a physician in recovery, a leader in his specialty. In relation to medical practice, he prides himself on his rationality, but he could only explain his sobriety as an act of faith: It was a "miracle" that the AA fellowship saved his career and family, even his life.

Our purpose here is to consider the words of such AA members and to examine research on addiction and recovery so that we can develop an understanding of how so many people achieve recovery from addiction through AA, and how others do not. As we do this, we will be getting a clear idea of what AA is, and the role it can play in helping people escape from the destructive effects of addiction.

Here is an example of the beginning of the kind of recovery that some AA members report. It shows how grave an addictive illness can become, and suggests a "spiritual renewal" that can sometimes precede an experience of redemption. This is what a public advocate for better treatment told me about the experience he had on his way into the fold of the AA fellowship:

> I'm in a detox on suicide watch, and I'm lying there, literally, on a rubber mat in the hallway in the detox unit where they can watch me. And I hear a whisper in my ear; it was St. Paul. That's all it was. I heard it; I know I heard it to the extent that it got me to take action. And yet there was nobody there. So it's not like somebody else whispered into my ear. And I considered that to be my spiritual awakening.

Such an experience is remarkable, and most people get engaged in AA in a more conventional way: They attend some meetings and begin to respond to the support of longer term members.

Federal surveys tell us that 3.4% of Americans have encountered Twelve Step groups at some time in their lives,[1] but such surveys cannot tell us what happened on the way to these encounters, and what kind of change might await some of these people if they decide to join. I would like to clarify that in this book.

I include many quotations here from patients of mine and from AA members with whom I have spoken. Their words have been modified very little, only to improve the syntax and clarity, and to preserve their anonymity. These quotations are not here just to illustrate the colorful way some AA members speak, but to convey the very personal and unique ways people experience their troubles and their recovery. Generalizations about the nature of addiction, many of them research-based, are valuable, and we will consider them, but they do not explain what can happen to a given person, because each person's story is unique. No one is merely part of a study population. Some of these people were at the end of their ropes, and others were just in bad trouble. Some chose to get better with help in AA; others did not.

There has been little available to the public, and even to health professionals, in explaining how AA "works." One might think that doctors could help by providing this for their patients, and could decide whether a given patient might benefit from AA. In fact, most all doctors, even addiction specialists, know less about this fellowship than one might think.

We *do* have a growing body of research on AA that shows how it can help in promoting people's recovery, and I have edited a dense volume with a colleague on these findings,[2] and I will draw on them here. But what we do not have is a book that captures the complexity of people's encounters with AA, both in their words and from clinical experience, with this backed up by a perspective based on research. I hope this book will address this need.

Many people know AA primarily from Hollywood. In one movie,[3] a studio executive is breezing along the freeway in his convertible and speaking on the phone. He says that he is going to an AA meeting. The retort at the other end of the line is, "But you're not an alcoholic." He answers, "That's where all the deals are made."

This may be true in cinematic Hollywood, but there is clearly more to it than that, even in Hollywood and on TV. Many people we know only from the media have gone to AA meetings because of *real* trouble—more than a compromised movie deal. Some of them, we hear, keep relapsing to alcohol and drugs, and their troubles are sensationalized and portrayed by paparazzi. But if they do "get better," they stop talking publicly about their experience in AA. In the fellowship's words, "Anonymity is the spiritual foundation of all our traditions . . ."[4] That is to say, one is not supposed to tout one's AA membership publicly. Fortunately, this has not prevented the AA members I will be citing here from sharing their experiences with us anonymously.

We often hear about AA when people tell about how someone they know had a bad addiction problem and got sober in AA. Or they can tell about an alcoholic relative who may have gone to AA, but never did get better. I hear this regularly from patients who come to me with an alcohol or drug problem; many of them can describe a relative who had a problem like their own, because alcoholism and drug problems so often run in families.

There are two million AA members worldwide about whom such stories can be told, because AA is so ubiquitous. No one is very far from a Twelve Step meeting anywhere in the States. Although the meetings are not announced with billboards, they can be located easily by plugging Alcoholics Anonymous or Narcotics Anonymous into the search engine of a computer. In the United States, there are over 60,000 weekly groups, and almost as many groups overseas. They are only a computer click away.

AA has become somewhat controversial, and there are a lot of misapprehensions that can leave an addicted person, a family member, or a therapist, too, unclear about its actual utility, and for whom it is appropriate. In fact, other than long-term AA members, few people are familiar with the basics of what membership entails, such as the way people get involved, what the Twelve Steps are understood to mean, and the role that experiences such as "spiritual awakening" play in the fellowship. Absent this, it is hard to make objective sense of what AA does or does not have to offer.

So then, for whom is this book written? First of all, it can help people with substance abuse problems who want to know whether and how AA might help them. Being told, "You need to go to AA," or just walking into an AA meeting on one's own, is like landing in a country that is very different from any visited before, and it can be daunting. A newcomer would wonder: "Is this for me? Why do they talk about God? How can it help with a problem I'm not even sure I have?"

Then there is the family member or friend who knows of no other option than to suggest AA to an addicted person. Maybe a doctor said to start a friend or spouse with AA, and may not have said much more. These people may even know someone in AA, but cannot quite figure out why they kept on going there for years. What are they doing in this group? Is it a cult?

Finally, health professionals need a book that gives them a coherent and objective sense of what this fellowship is like. Certainly, they cannot be of much help to their patients using a tool with which they themselves have no familiarity. Doctors would not want to employ a medication or a piece of equipment that they did not understand. Doesn't this apply to AA, too?

So this book is framed to explain what people are doing at those AA meetings, and what they are actually up to there. Here are some questions to be answered: Who is suitable for AA? What do AA sponsors do? What does AA's avowal of a higher power mean? What does the research show about whom it helps?

SO WHAT *IS* AA?

Here is some basic information about this fellowship to help the reader enter into this domain with some hold on what it is like. Alcoholics Anonymous dates back to 1935, at a time when there was no place for alcoholics to turn for help to relieve their compulsion to drink, except maybe a quest for religious transformation. A chronic alcoholic securities analyst, William Wilson, had experienced many failures in trying to stay sober. He would "dry out" with the help of doctors who meant well, but they had no way to help him from later relapsing. While in the hospital in New York one more time, he had a vision of a divine intervention, and vowed to not drink again. Some months after this, he was in Akron, Ohio on business, and was struggling to stay sober. He got together with a physician, Robert

Smith, and together they kept each other from relapsing into drinking. They then decided they would help other alcoholics do the same, Bill in New York and Dr. Bob in Akron.

Initially, they achieved little success in recruiting other drinkers, and the fellowship grew slowly. After ten years, though, it counted its membership at 13,000, and by 1950, almost 100,000. For the last twenty-five years, the membership has remained at about two million worldwide.[5] Extrapolating from these numbers, it appears that at any given time nowadays, an equal number of people are joining and moving on from the fellowship.

According to AA surveys, half of those attending have been sober for more than five years. They are a backbone for the organization, helping new attendees to get settled into the program. The survey also reveals that a large majority of members have come there either on their own or were referred by family or friends. We have surprisingly less research-based information about these members than one might think, because most all of the studies on AA have been done on the minority who were referred from treatment programs and other institutions.

There is a sequence to be taken on the AA path toward sobriety, primarily involving "working" the Twelve Steps: admitting powerlessness over alcohol, turning for help to a higher power (a somewhat flexible term in the program), acknowledging one's shortcomings, making amends, engaging in prayer and meditation, and helping other alcoholics. Most long-term members have followed these Steps with support from another member—a sponsor—whom they select for themselves. Committed members do "service" to help other alcoholics. This latter zealously felt mission has led the fellowship to extend its presence to 103 different countries, and its principal text, *Alcoholics Anonymous,* to sell many millions of copies.

AA, by the way, is a participatory democracy in that it is set up in a rather unique way. According to its operating principles, all AA groups are independent and self-governing. This is far from a typical corporate structure, which is how professional treatment programs are set up, where authority rests on a hierarchy that dictates how front-line operations run. This diffusion of control to the individual groups is notable in light of the consistency with which the various groups uphold AA's operating principles. The AA General Service Board, chosen by representatives from district committees and area assemblies, themselves elected by representatives of the local groups, just sets broad policy, which must then be approved by the elected conference members.

Because of its decentralization, the fellowship has virtually no budget except for a small number of employees in its central office. It relies on volunteers in the respective locales for answering phones to refer people to meetings and for disseminating pamphlets with consensus documents approved by its General Service Conference. However diffuse this may be, fidelity to the program's practices has been consistent and reliable across its many groups and countries. This is certainly evident in the meetings I have attended (as a non-alcoholic observer), in patients I have treated, and in those I have interviewed at length. There is no organization quite like it.

Some differences do exist between members. Some attend for years on end, but many who benefit from AA do not follow the steps, and benefit from attending a number of meetings nonetheless. They may not get a sponsor, but may achieve stability in sobriety based on their limited participation over time. One contemporary trend is that a large number of AA members have abused substances other than alcohol, everything from marijuana to prescription medication. This is an issue because some meetings do not welcome people addicted to drugs other than alcohol. In an effort to address this, the Twelve Steps were adopted by another similar organization, Narcotics Anonymous, which focuses on the many other drugs of abuse and has 50,000 groups worldwide.

The years since AA's inception have seen a great deal of progress in the treatment of addiction. Cognitive behavioral therapy that focuses on triggers for relapse has come to be employed by many therapists. Family treatments that focus on promoting support from people close to an addicted person have been widely accepted, and there are also large-scale programs like therapeutic communities and rehabilitation centers. Methadone, and more recently buprenorphine, were developed for people addicted to heroin and related narcotics, and there are also a number of medications used to promote decreased craving for alcohol. But participants in all of these approaches can benefit from experience with Twelve Step groups. This is particularly true for those dependent on drugs like cocaine and methamphetamine, and even marijuana and its synthetic congeners, for which we do not have pharmacologic treatments when someone's addiction becomes deeply rooted. The drugs people can get in trouble with have proliferated in recent years, in both number and nature. So even though new treatment options have been developed, in many respects, Twelve Step-based recovery is still a bulwark for many of those most severely disabled by addiction.

DIFFERENT PATHWAYS

People who come to AA each have had their own particular experiences, and anyone who wants to know what the fellowship can offer really needs to be apprised of the diversity of encounters that people report. A few examples of these illustrate this point. One patient I consulted on went to an AA meeting at my request, and came back flushed with euphoria from its congenial atmosphere; he found it to be exciting and engaging, but decided it was not for him. He was sure he could control his drinking, and kept it up, and continued to have ongoing trouble with his family. Another attended at times, but it was only after her collapse in remorse in a drinking binge because of trouble with a boyfriend that she decide to fully own up to her drinking. She began to take the AA program seriously and got sober. Another patient, long suffering from anxiety, agreed to attend, and found the members he met accepting and supportive. He continued to go with regularity, got a sponsor, and never drank again over the ensuing years. A college dropout addicted to pain pills graduated from rehab, agreeing to attend meetings, and did do so. He had a relapse after one month, and in a near panic rushed to a meeting and got a sponsor. That was the last he took pills or had a drink. Another patient attended AA for years, always struggling with relapses. Tragically, in the end she died of her illness from alcohol poisoning at a dose more than her body could sustain. A homeless, depressed man in our city hospital could not stop drinking, and was plagued by suicidal thoughts. When I asked him what kept him alive, he said it was the AA meetings he attended near Times Square, even though he could not stay sober.

So, some who enter into the fellowship will achieve sobriety with a relatively modest involvement, after attending meetings with some regularity for a time. Here is one man, compromised by his alcohol problem, but not to the degree of many of the more severely affected members, but who got sober while in therapy and going to two meetings a week:

> Not everybody goes in and finds sponsors; not everybody goes religiously. I'm sure that there are people who go religiously and work the Steps, and there are some who go religiously and don't work the Steps. I don't need to write down who I wronged while I was drinking, although generally, I've done some bad things. I did some bad things to myself, too, which upset me, but it wasn't that deeply damaging.

On the other hand, many members fully commit, and attend persistently for years on end, avowing that they would be vulnerable to relapse if they stopped. This is how one woman described this. Her long travail of destructive addiction had begun early in adolescence:

> A lot of people go out and pick up a drink, because I know; I relapsed. Sixteen years ago, five of my family members had died, all within a year. At my

stepfather's funeral, my cousins passed around a joint and I took a puff off of that joint. I never planned it; it just happened. Then I picked up a drink. It was very brief, but some horrible things happened, and I wasn't going to my [AA] meetings at the time. The biggest lesson I ever learned was that no, I can't go down that path again.

She was not going to take any more chances with her disease, and continued to attend regularly.

So what can someone anticipate about an AA encounter for a particular addicted person for whom they care? What can you, the reader, take with you that will afford you an understanding of this unique fellowship, to see how it might fit into the life of such a person? Or, what if you are a healthcare professional who wants to understand how this most successful volunteer organization of the last hundred years can help your patients?

To answer these questions, to give you a basis for making a judgment, you do need to be introduced to AA through the experience of people who have encountered it, and who have described the complex and varied paths they followed. A discussion of what we have discovered from research that sheds light on it is also required. All this information needs to be organized in a systematic way. This is what this book sets out to do. I will try to do this along with a discussion of the nature of the disease of addiction it addresses. The book will address how AA arose and operates; the psychology of how people become engaged; and the stages they pass through as prescribed by the fellowship. We will, as well, consider a biologic perspective, based on contemporary research, on how AA prayers can alter the very craving for alcohol that members must escape. We also will cover particular studies that shed light on the outcome of membership; and finally, we will examine some alternative or complementary options that a substance-abusing person can pursue in seeking help.

PART I

Alcoholics Anonymous in the Public Arena

CHAPTER 1

Its Origin and Evolution

Every AA member who reads the fellowship's literature knows of the spark that ignited this worldwide movement. It happened one day in 1934 as Bill W, AA's cofounder, was struggling to escape the suffering of his years of uncontrolled drinking. He later recounted that, in his misery, he lay in his hospital bed despairing of relief:

> All at once I found myself crying out, "If there is a God, let him show himself! I am ready to do anything, anything!" Suddenly the room lit up with a great white light. I was caught up in an ecstasy which there are not words to describe. It seemed to me, in my mind's eye, that I was on a mountain and that a wind not of air but of spirit was blowing. And it burst upon me that I was a free man. Slowly the ecstasy subsided. I lay there on the bed, but now for a time I was in another world, a new world of consciousness . . . and I thought to myself, "So this is the God of the preachers!" A great peace stole over me.[1]

AA certainly was not an inevitable result of this event. We can look further to see how this remarkably successful worldwide network for recovery ensued from Bill's spiritual experiences, and we can begin by considering his own story.

THE BEGINNINGS OF ALCOHOLICS ANONYMOUS

William Wilson (1895–1971) was a securities analyst living in New York, whose depression early in life contributed to his falling into heavy drinking. In 1934, Bill W, as he came to be known in AA, was in utter despair.

His alcoholism had driven him to bingeing for days, suffering extensive blackouts, and even stealing money from his wife—all this leading him to multiple hospital stays for drying out. On his way to his fourth such episode, he drank four beers, and then admitted himself to the Town Hospital in upper Manhattan. As we saw, he would ultimately describe the sudden startling and transcendent experience he had while in his hospital room.

Bill was uncertain of what it meant, but his doctor told him that it was not a sign of the insanity he feared, but rather a religious experience. Bill saw this as a turning point and decided, with great conviction, that he would never drink again. He began attending a religious revivalist program, the Oxford Group, which espoused the idea that the problems of the world could be healed by members' personal spiritual change, thereby promoting a spiritual awakening among involved members.

Several months later, Bill, still not drinking, was on a business trip in Akron, Ohio, and was struggling to stay sober. He was introduced to a physician, Dr. Bob, who also was trying to achieve sobriety and participating in the Oxford Group. The two men banded together, spent days supporting each other, and established a bond that would later be viewed as the founding of AA, in 1935.

Over the ensuing months, the two became aware that they themselves could embark on a project directed at men who would support each other in abstinence. It had no Steps at the time, and no rules other than, "Don't Drink." Bill returned home, and now their initiative had two homes, one in Akron and one in New York. He and Bob began enlisting new members in a fledgling fellowship, and soon emerged from under the umbrella of the Oxford Group. As Bill later explained, "The Oxford Group wanted to save the world, and I only wanted to save drunks." In actuality, he and Bob became unwelcome in the Oxford Group because they were so preoccupied with alcoholism.[2]

By 1938, the Twelve Steps were being formulated, and Bill began putting together the book, *Alcoholics Anonymous*, that later gave the movement its name. Its first part conveyed the AA philosophy and program, and this was followed by chapters recounting the experiences of early members. The membership now had reached one hundred, and Bill succeeded in raising money for the book's publication. It was most heartening that it was reviewed in *The New York Times*, but despite this and the enthusiasm of early members, sales of the book were modest.

The exact nature of what the fledgling fellowship was did not initially emerge with clarity. Consideration was given to it operating residential programs for rehabilitation, and of including professional roles, with salaried members. John D. Rockefeller was strongly supportive of the AA concept, but whether out of parsimony or vision, he refused to provide major support and, much to the dismay of Bill, would not underwrite the program. Ironically, the absence of substantial external fiscal support was instrumental in shaping AA into a fully nonprofessional, volunteer organization, with no residences—a format central to its later success. By 1941, newspaper articles, including one in the nationally popular *Saturday Evening Post*, generated interest in AA. By the end of that year, the fellowship counted some 8,000 members.[3]

ORIGINS IN AMERICAN CULTURE

In many respects, AA was very much a product of the American society and culture from which it arose. Some of the original British colonies were founded because of the need for escape from the control of European religious authorities, and the country was framed as an organized polity by its Founding Fathers, many of whom, like Thomas Jefferson and Benjamin Franklin, were Deists. That is to say, they believed in the existence of a Creator, but eschewed the idea of organized religion with its literal belief in scriptures and miracles, and the need for a clergy to communicate the Creator's will. The Virginia Statute for Religious Freedom,[4] drafted by Thomas Jefferson, illustrated this: "Almighty God hath created the mind free" and "no man shall be compelled to frequent or support any religious worship, place, or ministry whatsoever." This concept of religious liberty, free of an alliance between the state and a given religious denomination was entrenched in the country's Bill of Rights. This view of a nondenominational higher power was easily compatible with the one cited in the Twelve Steps.

Other developments closer to AA's inception also supported this concept. The late nineteenth century saw a broadening of ideas beyond traditional Christian doctrine. This derived in part from a growing acquaintance with Eastern religions such as Hinduism and Buddhism, which differed from a Christian outlook. Eventually, the acquaintance came to be expressed in a seventeen-day conference, the Parliament of the World's Religions, held in Chicago in 1893. This conclave was established in an attempt to create a global dialogue among faiths, with representatives of both Eastern and Western religious traditions. This diversity also promoted a nondogmatic conception of religious thinking, one that would further augment the theme of nondenominational belief in a Creator.

Other religious traditions were relevant as well. The American culture had evangelical strains that emerged in two Great Awakenings over the course of the country's early history, and AA's character was similar to an evangelical movement, but not quite a religious one. The issue of religion was always ambivalently felt. After the Steps were framed, the word "God" was later set to be followed by the phrase "as we understood Him," leaving a member the latitude to accede to an ill-defined Higher Power rather than follow a traditional deity. Nonetheless, *Alcoholics Anonymous*, often called the "Big Book," written under Bill's supervision and published in 1939, did reflect the intensity of religious feelings of early members. It included two prayers, the first beginning with, "God, I offer myself to Thee—to build with me and to do with me as Thou wilt," and the second with, "My Creator, I am now willing that you should have all of me, good and bad." Although not rigidly defined, the Higher Power was often understood to be the recipient of personalized devotion.

A more generic view of AA's spiritual renewal appeared in an appendix in later editions. It cited William James, a physician and professor at Harvard, who taught what is thought to be the first psychology course in the United States. He expressed the view that religion and spirituality were inherent in human nature. His classic 1902 book, *The Varieties of Religious Experience*,[5] spelled out two types of spiritual renewal. One was self-surrender, a relatively passive experience like that of Bill W. The second, the volitional type, takes place when individuals decide that they wish to make spiritual changes in their lives. This latter experience is described as the type of spiritual renewal encountered by most AA members, and as being "of the educational variety, developing over time."[6]

THE TWELVE TRADITIONS

Bill knew that AA as an organization had to have consensually accepted principles of operation. In the 1940s, he began preparing AA's Twelve Traditions to frame the fellowship's governing principles. In many ways, they are central to why the fellowship has been so successful in holding together while spreading widely. Bill wrote of his travail in getting the Traditions accepted, reporting that "people were at first politely attentive, though it must be confessed that some did go to sleep during my early harangues. But after a while, I got letters containing sentiments like this: '. . . for heaven's sake, please don't talk anymore about those blasted traditions!.'"[7] He persisted nonetheless. In 1944, AA developed a newsletter, *The Grapevine*, which over the years has come to serve as a vehicle for publishing its deliberations and policies. The Twelve Traditions first appeared there two years after the newsletter was established.

Here are some key aspects of the Traditions: "Our leaders are but trusted servants; they do not govern. . . . Each group should be autonomous, except in matters affecting other groups or AA as a whole." This has yielded a unique structure to the fellowship, wherein all AA groups operate independently but do send representatives to higher levels of governance to formulate policy. As the fellowship grew, these levels of governance came to operate through a series of elected bodies, district committees that elect area assemblies. At the General Service Conference, the membership of a General Service Board is affirmed. This Board frames general policy but does not have authority over any of the groups' operation. Elected officials are, therefore, "trusted servants" rather than managers. All this represents an adaptation of an American democratic culture. Notably, the General Service Board is the only entity within the fellowship's governance where there is typically a formal role for non-alcoholics. Of the Board's twenty-one members, seven positions are allocated to non-alcoholics.

The Twelve Traditions serve to protect the fellowship from outside intrusion. Here are some more of them: "Each group has but one primary purpose—to carry its message to the alcoholic who still suffers. . . . An AA group ought never endorse, finance or lend the AA name to any related facility or outside enterprise, lest problems of money, property and prestige divert us from our primary purpose." This has assured that over the years, despite the emergence of many worthwhile medical and social movements, as well as new psychological and medical treatments, the fellowship has avoided internal strife by eschewing promotion of other causes or treatments, however worthwhile they may be. AA policy today is that members' medical treatment and medications are a matter determined between them and their doctors. This has served to counter (usually effectively) the bias that many members have expressed over treatments such as antidepressants, now taken by many who attend the meetings. Such a policy keeps medication issues out of the meetings.

Furthermore, "Our public relations policy is based on attraction rather than promotion; we need always maintain personal anonymity at the level of press, radio and films." This ensures that AA will not make itself a focus of advertising or sought-after publicity. It does not run membership campaigns or allow members to use AA membership to achieve personal recognition. Furthermore, "Anonymity is the spiritual foundation of all our Traditions, ever reminding us to put principles above personalities." This provides assurance that a person can appear at meetings and speak freely without fear of public exposure. It also means that people attending AA cannot use the fact of their membership to personal advantage. Furthermore, whether in TV appearances or in memoirs, members are not seen publicly touting their participation in AA. What this has resulted in, in practice, is that AA members may openly discuss medical contributions to their recovery, but do not typically detail their AA experience. This is why many prominent people in Twelve-Step recovery talk about their new well-being, but do not explicitly say what AA did for them. Ironically, it also means that public testimony of the benefit people get from AA is limited. Often, criticism of AA gets more media attention than discussion of its benefits.

The fellowship was still very much an instrument of Bill's charisma in its early decades. Its gradual transformation into a functioning organization can be considered by recourse to a model described by the sociologist Max Weber, who developed a way of understanding the evolution of religious and similarly intensely held movements,[8] and who described how charismatic leadership evolves. Weber defined charismatic leaders as having exceptional qualities that attract people to them and to what they stand for. Bill's role in shaping the way AA achieved its growth and the members' response to him as time went on reflected this unique quality. Bill realized, however, that the fellowship could not rest on the shoulders of one person and his leadership. If the legacy of charisma is to persist, Weber pointed out, it must be "routinized," or invested in some sort of bureaucratic structure that inherits its leader's "sacred" mantle. Bill intuitively was determined to see this happen through framing the Twelve Traditions. Then he followed them with the Twelve Concepts for World Service, adopted by AA's General Services Conference in 1962. These framed the guidelines for how the fellowship would be organized and operated, and institutionalized the democratically elected General Service Board. Importantly, the Concepts invested "final responsibility" in the "collective conscience of [the] whole Fellowship." The latter commitment represents both a strength and perhaps a weakness. It means that the fellowship does not splinter based on differing factions, because no minority opinion can be over-ridden by the majority. On the other hand, it can impede progress when conservative members block development of new, potentially useful, initiatives. Altogether, though, Bill's influence in framing the Traditions and Concepts is what has helped AA to survive and flourish. It is for this reason that the author Aldous Huxley, who lived to see the fruit of Bill's efforts, called him "the greatest social architect of our century."

As an aside, Bill was far from perfect in some of his personal relations. Although his marriage lasted fifty-three years until his death in 1971, his wife Lois suffered greatly over the years due to his repeated flirtations and womanizing during the forties, fifties, and sixties[9] while AA was being successfully established.

The number of members in AA is documented in the fellowship's early literature and the reports of their triennial surveys. These are informative because they can give us an understanding of the fellowship's evolution and its current status. At its inception in 1935, there were two members, Bill W and Dr. Bob. Two years later in 1937, there were forty members; ten years after that there were 40,000 members; and ten years later there were over 100,000 members. This clearly represented a period of dramatic growth. During these years there were hardly any resources for an alcoholic to turn to for support in recovery, and given the zeal of the members at that time, this growth is understandable. But the following decade up to 1967 saw an expansion of membership of only 50%. Since 1990, the membership has actually been flat at about two million. Since the nineties, the ratio between the membership and the overall population has not increased, just hovered around 0.4%. One might say that over this last generation the portion of the population who were likely to join AA has stabilized. After all, there has to be some limit to the number of alcoholics, and for that matter, some drug addicts, too, who are likely to want to join.[10]

What does this portend for the future? The fellowship seems to be able to keep its penetration of the "available market" stable, but the more recent availability for accessing other options for achieving recovery may be limiting further growth. Professionals have entered the field of addiction treatment in increasing numbers over recent decades, with social workers, psychologists, and psychiatrists providing treatment that is supportive of recovery. What may not have become influential as of yet, are medications that might make a significant dent in the outcome of treatment. These could move the recovery process forward in some measure. Naltrexone, the most commonly prescribed medication for suppressing craving for alcohol, has on average not been shown in controlled studies to have a remarkably greater effect than a contrasting placebo pill. (Although it has been found helpful for some people.) What this boils down to is that most patients on this drug do not achieve a major decrease in the likelihood of them returning to heavy drinking.[11] This can be put statistically in the following way: In order to achieve getting one patient on naltrexone to avoid returning to heavy drinking, twelve patients would have to be treated overall. Although this does represent a beneficial effect, its limited impact makes it understandable that many of the clinics treating alcoholic people do not invest much effort in applying this pharmacologic option.

Altogether, therefore, one can say that at present there seems to be a relatively stable portion of the population who are AA members at any given time. Most of them are likely persons with serious alcohol problems who need the committed membership in the fellowship to maintain their abstinence. Could these long-term members remove themselves from AA and still stay free of highly compromising drinking patterns? Perhaps some could, and some do, but no one is about to press long-term AA members to jettison their participation in the hope that things would work out well.

CHAPTER 2
Controversies

Alcoholics Anonymous has 100,000 regular group meetings and over two million members worldwide, and is recognized among the public as a principal resource for addicted people to turn to for recovery. Recent years, however, have brought on numerous critiques of AA, and questions about whether it does, indeed, offer the benefits that some members avow. Here are three controversial issues that are regularly brought up about it.

QUESTIONS ABOUT GOD AND A HIGHER POWER

AA designates itself as a "spiritual fellowship," and its writings are infused with the concept of God, or a Higher Power. In fact, six of its Twelve Steps mention God, sometimes "as we understood Him," or just as "a Power greater than ourselves." There is a history behind the role of the God concept, one certainly related to the American culture of the early twentieth century, where the role of God in people's lives was taken by most as a matter of fact. At that time Bill W, the cofounder of AA, had attended meetings of the Oxford Group before the revelation that led him to lifelong abstinence. In that setting, oriented to a Christian concept of commitment to God, he had to pledge his life to Christ; and four "practices" of the Oxford Group were later influential in his development of AA's Twelve Steps.

The first edition of AA's Big Book, *Alcoholics Anonymous*,[1] with notations from Bill himself, is revealing. The notes reflect an attempt to make the program more acceptable to people who were not devout Christians, thus the terms "Higher Power" and "God *as we understood him*" were ultimately used instead of "Jesus Christ," which was originally in the text. The

Seventh AA Step was also softened, by deleting, "Humbly, on our knees, ask Him to remove our shortcomings—holding nothing back"—a phrase that evoked Christian worship. This became "Humbly ask Him to remove our shortcomings." The Big Book also includes an option of traditional prayer: "God, I offer myself to Thee—to build within me and to do to me as Thou will . . ." But this is preceded by, "Many of us said to our Maker, *as we understood him.*"[2] This serves as a preface to allow for members who are not among the "many."

One may ask whether AA is a religious fellowship or just a spiritual one. Although it designates itself as "spiritual," there is a problem in terms of how one discriminates between attitudes or activities that can be called spiritual and those that could be called religious. Religion is an organized system of beliefs and rituals associated with a sense of transcendence. Generally, but not always, there is a commitment to a specific entity, such as a Higher Power or a God. Spirituality, on the other hand, can be understood more broadly as that which gives the person meaning and purpose in life. It *can* be expressed in religious observance, but can also refer to commitment to higher ideals, and can connect a community of people with a larger philosophical outlook. In contrast to religion, spirituality is not necessarily something one can clearly see in action, given that there are usually no formal rituals. Admittedly, for AA, it may be hard to distinguish between the two, because AA does have some rituals and does recognize a Higher Power. Whatever the case, AA members are quick to say that their movement is not a religion, which actually makes sense.

All this can have practical implications. For one thing, legally, there is an issue of whether someone can be told to attend a Twelve Step-based treatment program, which some do say is inherently religious in nature. What has been established in legal proceedings is that private treatment programs, like most rehabs, can require attendance at AA meetings, but governmental ones, like a parole system or the Veterans Health Administration (VA), are constrained from doing so, because of the constitutionally derived separation of church and state. A governmental agency must offer alternatives when a person (e.g., a parolee) asks for them.

Here is another issue: Are statements made at Twelve Step meetings protected by confidentiality, as they would be if they were made to a priest or minister? Here again legal proceedings ensued when a case arose where someone had spoken at an AA meeting about having committed a murder, and the information was later brought to the attention of authorities. Because of technicalities, a final decision in case law on this was never formally settled, so the issue remains unresolved.

The confidentiality issue can become fodder for Hollywood, as was highlighted in the movie, "You Kill Me" (2007). Frank, an alcoholic hit man, played by Ben Kingsley, is sent from the East Coast mob to San Francisco to "get his act together" and deal with his alcoholism. At one AA meeting there, he describes his vocation, and says he wants to be free of his drinking problem so he can move on with his career as a hit man. The attendees were understandably nonplussed. Frank does achieve sobriety, moves on, and has to commit one more killing, "justified" in mob terms.

Back to the Big Book: One chapter, "We Agnostics," points out that "about half of the original fellowship" consisted of atheists or agnostics, and then goes on to give advice as to how such members can find "a Power greater than ourselves." It reassures the reader that "faith in some kind of God was a part of our make-up, just as much as the feeling we have for a friend. Sometimes we had to search fearlessly, but He was there . . . We found the Great Reality deep down within us."[3] I will have more to say about this in the chapter that describes a model for AA based on social neuroscience. In brief, though, we can characterize, even physiologically, how such a shared conception of God can exist within members' minds.

In trying to capture how people grapple with this issue, I asked members what spirituality and the concept of a Higher Power meant to them. Let's consider how one person, with twenty years of sobriety but no religious orientation, was able to reconcile herself to the role of God in AA, as she described her spirituality in AA:

> Quit thinking that it's out there. It's something that you have to feel, not if you're good enough, if you're smart enough, if you talk loud enough. I think that somehow God or a Higher Power has shown His face to me in the people I have known in AA, because I have been more open to it. That's what has made me feel very much a spiritual connection. So somehow that feeling, like I was led by my Higher Power to stay sober—there has to be something at work. I have a hard time with a lot of organized religion, but I feel that this is a very different thing. It's a spiritual connection to a Higher Power or to God . . . "It doesn't matter who your Higher Power is as long as it isn't you"—if it has to be the group, if it has to be something—whatever it is that keeps you coming.

DOES AA OVERPROMISE?

In one section of its text, *Alcoholics Anonymous,* that has remained unchanged since 1939, it appears that AA may overstate what it can do for an alcoholic:

> Rarely have we seen a person fail who has thoroughly followed our path. Those who do not recover are people who cannot or will not completely give themselves to this simple program, usually men and women who are constitutionally incapable of being honest with themselves. They are such unfortunates.[1]

Admittedly, this sounds a bit grandiose and self-congratulatory, but let's considers it from both a historical and a clinical perspective. When AA's Big Book first appeared, the early members saw it as a singular option for the chronic alcoholic to achieve sobriety. At that time, the assumption made by many in the AA circle was that alcoholism represented a grave and inevitable downhill course for those who continued to drink. So it came to be that the instruction many long-term members gave to new recruits was to make "90 meetings in 90 days." One might well conclude that for those recruits who committed themselves to that degree of involvement, the likelihood of success was considerable. But in some ways this was a tautology, which is to say, this was needlessly self-fulfilling, in that most any person who could bring themselves to meet this expectation was likely to become committed to a course of recovery in the program. Does that mean that others should be considered "incapable of being honest with themselves?"

I have found that patients who commit to regular AA attendance along the lines I prescribe do, indeed, do well. My own approach is to ask them to go to two or three meetings a week at first, because many have busy schedules and are not likely to find it possible to do more than this. I also have them keep a record of the meetings they attended, which we review together in our sessions. This is done along with ongoing therapy.

But what about those who are "constitutionally incapable of being honest with themselves?" This can be considered from a psychological perspective. Karen was a mother of two whose husband, successful in business, was committed to the marriage but regularly critical of her. Karen drank too much, and by the time she saw me she was having trouble at home. She did keep the house in relative order, and had done a journeyman job in raising their two boys as young children. But recently, with the boys in their teens, her husband would come home to find her intoxicated, and not in great shape to manage their household.

So Karen came to see me at her husband's behest, and for a long time, at her request, I tried to help her move toward controlling her level of drinking. This never worked, and the drinking got worse. So we turned to AA, and Karen did a reasonable job attending the meetings, but could never bring herself to accept the fact that she had to stop drinking. In fact, she continued to go downhill, appearing at a PTA meeting visibly intoxicated, and with slurred speech. The story went on from there with her involvement on and off in AA and with two stints in rehab. Each time she left rehab intending to go to community-based AA meetings, but suffering a continuing decline in her drinking status. Ultimately, she had to settle in a sober living residential community for three months before finally reaching an accommodation to sobriety.

Had Karen been constitutionally incapable of being "honest with herself?" She was inherently a passive woman, never having been able to stabilize a career or assert herself with her husband. Over time it became clear that drinking was a part of her identity as her own (self-defeating) way of asserting her autonomy. She could not stand up to her husband, or even her friends. The craving, the compulsion to drink, had not been that severe, but even though the consequences of her drinking became increasingly compromising, she could not acknowledge that she had to give up that seeming island of autonomy.

The irrationality behind this was evident during one part of her ongoing and rocky treatment when she had enrolled in a social work training program and encountered clients with drinking problems like hers. I would ask her what she would tell such a person about sobriety, and she said that she would tell them that they had to stop drinking—but she refused to acknowledge the fact that she herself could not drink. This was an example of the nature of denial (dishonesty with themselves, as it were) that can afflict some alcoholics, and which can be an impediment moving forward.

Then what can we say about the many people for whom AA is beneficial?

Does it work? This is a complicated question, about which more will be discussed in a separate chapter on AA's effectiveness, but we can consider this question now in light of controversies about the fellowship's effectiveness. After all, AA is an approach that was not developed on the basis of clinical research, but emerged instead as a way that lay people came to manage their own alcoholism. Because AA membership is anonymous, its members cannot be systematically followed up for evaluation. Given the medical community's reliance on randomized, controlled trials for validation, there is no structured research on AA that meets this criterion. This is not the way we test the effectiveness of new treatments nowadays. Rather, we assign various therapies or drugs at random against alternative treatments.

This means there is no easy way to rebut the critiques of some researchers that AA is a folk remedy, rather than a valid approach to recovery. This critique was illustrated even forty years ago in an article in the *American Journal of Psychiatry*, the official scientific publication of the American

Psychiatric Association. It described AA as a craft handed down from one mentor to another, never scientifically validated, and not subject to improvements based on innovation coming from research. The authors' observation of AA-based therapists in alcohol clinics was that their attitudes were incompatible with those of the science-based clinicians who might work there.[2] Back then, in fact, there was little communication between AA-oriented clinical staff, mostly in Twelve-Step-based recovery, and staff doctors, who were often kept at arm's length. Integration has moved a long way since then in most, but not all, settings.

This questioning of AA was bolstered by a report prepared by the Cochrane Collaboration,[3] a system for evaluating medical treatments that concluded, "The available experimental studies did not demonstrate the effectiveness of AA or other 12-Step approaches in reducing alcohol use and achieving abstinence compared to other treatments . . . more efficacy studies are needed."

A principal resource on which the Cochrane report was based was a large-scale federal study, Project MATCH, designed in the 1990s to see whether certain alcoholics could be better matched with certain specific treatments rather than others. (Even $27 million later, they did not come up with a positive answer.)[4] Although Twelve Step Facilitation, a therapy designed to encourage alcoholics to go to AA, had been only recently developed, the academic researchers who prepared this study added it to the mix. Some expected that it would be of limited benefit. As a matter of fact, patients treated with this approach did as well as ones who were treated in experimentally designed treatments and, in fact, achieved a somewhat higher degree of abstinence by the end of the study follow-up.[5]

The longest follow-up study that can shed light on AA's efficacy was carried out by a research team from Stanford University.[6] They repeatedly contacted people over time who had sought treatment for alcoholism in community-based referral services. In the first year of follow-up, 59% of respondents entered professional treatment, and 58% entered AA. These folks were followed up for a full sixteen years, and the duration of AA attendance mediated 33% of the rates of abstinence; that is to say, it was a strong contributor to the likelihood of abstinence. In fact, for those who were in treatment during the first six months, later AA attendance was more associated with a positive outcome than was further treatment.

One psychiatrist has written that AA offers a comforting veneer of change, but that studies peg the success rate of AA somewhere between 5% and 10%, no better than rates of spontaneous remission.[7] What does this "success rate" of only 5% to 10% actually mean? The figure was based on a study that drew on data provided by AA itself in its surveys.[8] It was based on all those who first showed up at a meeting, no doubt many of them reluctant or pressured by family. Only 19% were still attending AA at one month, 10% at three months, and 5% at one year. But what this means is that for those who were still attending a month after first showing up, 52% were still attending at three months, and 26% after a year. That is to say, half of the people who are still showing up after three months were likely to be in attendance at the end of the year. In practical terms, this is as good as any of our other treatments for alcoholism. And this early figure included people who were not necessarily in professional treatment, but just showing up at a meeting. Nowadays some half of the people who first attend AA are being referred by a physician or other professional and are in some form of continuing care, in which they typically are encouraged to go to AA meetings. This materially bolsters the fellowship's effectiveness.

HOW ABOUT TREATMENT PROGRAMS AND REHABS?

One study is notable as a natural experiment. The largest network of alcohol (and drug) programs in the United States is the sprawling VA system. I first encountered it in framing a plan for dealing with the dually diagnosed (with substance abuse and mental illness) at the behest of New York State's Commissioner of Mental Health. Articles had been written years back about the Coatesville VA in Pennsylvania in the 1960s and 1970s, where chronic alcoholic vets could live in peace, absent an effective recovery-oriented treatment program. In time, though, the VA system has moved toward setting up active treatment units and clinics across the country. Given these programs, one could consider the outcome for patients in many locations.

Rudolf Moos at Stanford spearheaded much of this effort.[9] His team undertook a comparison of substance abuse treatments in a large number of VA programs, ones that were at liberty to apply whatever format they chose, based on the inclination of staff and program leadership. Some programs had an AA orientation while others adopted a more research-based approach, like cognitive behavior therapy. After two years, patients who were treated in the programs that had a Twelve Step orientation had higher rates of abstinence (50%) than those who were treated with the experimentally based cognitive-behavioral therapy (37%).[10] Although this was not a controlled study with prior randomization, it does offer a useful perspective on the utility of the Twelve Step approach when applied in an actual community-based setting.

On the other hand, many "rehab" programs that employ the Twelve Step approach appear to be cozy "spas" rather than serious healing centers. They may be publicized because they often treat celebrities who have made headlines with their alcohol- or drug-infused displays of bad behavior. Some are on beachfront settings where most anyone would want to vacation. Others feature "equine therapy," where you can develop a relationship with horses, as might the children of the wealthy. This can cast a shadow over AA's image as a means of rebuilding integrity and character in abstinence.

There is indeed a marked diversity in quality and mode of operation of the residential rehab programs that have emerged in recent years, and this field has a long way to go before the seriousness and competency of the best programs set the tone for the other ones. One analysis however, was done on patients completing treatment at the Hazelden Foundation hospital,[11] among the best established and most sophisticated of such Twelve Step-based residential rehabilitation settings. They reported a 53% rate of abstinence among those patients after one year of treatment, and an additional 45% had a substantially reduced rate of alcohol use. These figures were based on a careful follow-up, and corroborated by people like family or friends, who knew the status of the patients surveyed.

Altogether, research does suggest that AA, when combined with professional treatment, can provide a positive outcome. It can do well, not as a "treatment" in itself, but rather as a valuable component of a professionally framed program. This stipulation is actually the perspective put forth by the leading medical addiction treatment societies in the United States. So today, forward-looking rehabilitation programs, some now connected with university-affiliated medical centers, do rely on Twelve Step involvement for their patients. They also include professional therapy, and where indicated by contemporary standards of care, medications, too.

Admittedly, however, there are residential rehabs that are not among the most forward-looking or medically sophisticated, and there are people who go to AA who would benefit from professional treatment along with AA, but who do not have easy access to it. More and better standards of care are needed. The medical societies do provide extensive and ongoing training for their members for dealing with the complexities of addiction rehabilitation, and expect them to continue training as part of ongoing membership. Within this training there are a variety of approaches to effective addiction treatment, and the use of AA is certainly important among them.

SO, CONTROVERSY PERSISTS

The appeal of medications as an ideal, not just as a practical everyday solution, has given some clinical researchers an attractive alternative to the need for mutual help. In the end, this can come down to a matter of ideology, as expressed in two contrasting cultures. One looks to biological medicine as a solution, the other to a people-based approach, AA in particular.

Here is an example of how it plays out. Advocates of medications can write pointedly about the need to adopt naltrexone, the most widely prescribed medication for treating alcoholism.[12] But a review of all the studies on this medication finds that statistically, across studies, the large majority will return to heavy drinking.[13] Ironically, this is not unlike what has been said about the number of people who stick to AA for the first month. Yet, one leading researcher on medications for alcoholism has pointedly questioned the benefit of AA either "inside or outside a rehab facility."[14]

On the other hand, a group of physician specialists in addiction treatment, many of them who achieved recovery in Twelve Step programs, have banded together under the label "Like Minded Docs." They point out that AA and nonpharmacologic approaches are often given short shrift in the medical societies for addiction treatment, and they have tried to promote more attention to people-based recovery support. There is no doubt some validity to the concerns expressed in both camps.

IS ADDICTION A DISEASE?

AA certainly thinks so: "We are convinced to a man that alcoholics of our type are in the grip of a progressive illness."[1] This has appeared in each of the editions of *Alcoholics Anonymous* since 1939. Although AA grappled with the question, many people are ambivalent about this because it is hard to acknowledge that a behavior that looks like it could be controlled can be designated as a disease. The "disease concept," however, has become part of AA lore, having been influential in giving alcoholics the opportunity to relieve the burden of guilt for their actions through rejuvenation within the fellowship. In the decades since the mid-twentieth century, this conception has come to be elaborated in ways that impinge on how we understand recovery in the fellowship. To best understand AA's place in the contemporary culture, we need to look at how all this evolved.

Drinking too much alcohol was for the longest time considered by many in the public to be a choice with dubious moral taint, but in 1956, the American Medical Association declared that alcoholism *is* a disease, and therefore, merits medical intervention. But the ambivalence about the disorder has persisted. For example, the 1968 edition of the diagnostic lexicon of the American Psychiatric Association (APA), the *Diagnostic and Statistical Manual of Mental Disorders II*,[2] did include alcoholism and drug dependence among the mental disorders. Significantly though, it listed it under the category of personality disorders, which suggests that it reflects a defect in one's character, implicitly carrying a value judgment. In retrospect, it may also be somewhat embarrassing for the psychiatric profession that alcohol and drug dependence was listed right after sexual deviations (including homosexuality, which was later rescinded as a disease entity by the APA). Now, however, substance use disorders have their own section.

More recent enlightenment on this issue is characterized by a model put forward by Tom McLellan and colleagues in the *Journal of the American Medical Association* in 2000.[3] They defined alcohol and drug dependence as a chronic illness. They made the point that a careful review of the medical literature leads to likening dependencies to alcohol and drugs to chronic diseases like Type II diabetes, hypertension, and asthma, and they went through a careful review of the similarities among these illnesses in causes, consequences, and response to treatments. Regarding the origin of the illnesses, each is affected by both genetic and environmental factors; each has physical ill effects, each is subject to reduced consequences based on whether the afflicted person adheres to a prescribed medical treatment, and each is subject to relapse if the afflicted person does not adhere. The point here is also that none of these illnesses can be treated solely by responding to their acute symptoms; instead they require strategies for long-term care and proper medical management.

Let's for the moment consider the experience of two women who illustrate the innate and pernicious nature of this illness. Both were successful in their careers and motivated to have a good life, but fell prey to the ravages of alcohol, having been engulfed by the disease because of innate vulnerabilities that they could not master. One cannot help but think that they suffered a disease over which they had little control.

The first was the daughter of a chronic alcoholic. She forswore drinking all through her college years, but then came to New York and began hanging out with a group of people who drank socially, and sometimes quite heavily. She soon decided that she could join in, intending to do so in moderation, but quickly fell into a pattern of severe alcohol dependence, losing track of how she could limit her drinking, often blacking out, sometimes unsure of how or when she got home. She came to AA after one night of heavy drinking, having called a friend and despairingly asked if he thought she was an alcoholic, saying that, "Well if I'm not, I'm going off the roof. I just thought the other alternative is that I'm just plain crazy."

The second woman, previously a moderate social drinker, also collapsed into alcoholism, in her case after the breakup of her marriage. She was despairing of her future, having moved overseas from the States on the expectation that her husband would find some stability in his career with a new job opportunity. She had now sacrificed her own career, but soon realized that her husband was failing at holding a job. She then experienced aggravation of a chronic, anxious state. She also precipitously fell into severe drinking, ending up, over four years, with two bouts of rehab and numerous stays in emergency rooms because of the quantities she consumed. She was finally hospitalized with acute pancreatitis after appearing in an emergency room vomiting blood.

Two cases do not make a syndrome, but they illustrate how the seeds of this chronic illness may be lying fallow until they are given the chance to grow wildly and precipitously. Such cases suggest that many alcoholics (but not necessarily all) suffer the "allergy" to alcohol that AA came to use as a metaphor for an innate vulnerability to illness. For the first woman, this came about in the absence of any other apparent psychiatric problems. For the second, it was driven in part by an aggravation of her chronic anxiety.

There is another side to this story on alcoholism, however, one clearly not associated with the profound, likely biologically grounded, vulnerability that was evident in the lives of these two women. It relates to the role of a lifetime of heavy drinking that is seen as "normal" in a national culture, and the consequences of this for its population. This became apparent to me when traveling through the Soviet Union some years before the collapse of the Berlin Wall. I began my trip by reading an introduction to the country in the book, "The Russians,"[4] by a journalist who wrote about medical students being conscripted by the state to harvest crops in remote communes where the drunkenness was so pervasive that the local residents were incapable of effectively carrying out the work themselves. Upon arrival in Russia, I often saw men staggering in the streets, quite obviously drunk. As my family and I drove through the hinterland, we came across a factory. I looked in on the dining room at lunch time and the only nourishment one could see was either beer or hard liquor.

This aspect of Russian national culture goes back some centuries. In 1591, for example, the English ambassador to the court of Ivan the Terrible pointed out how important liquor tax revenue was to the state. He wrote that this long-standing issue would inevitably be sustained by the government's economic needs.[5] And so it has been, even on through the Soviet years. Lenin objected to this reliance on alcohol revenues, and banned vodka during the early years of the Soviet Union, only to have the ban lifted by Stalin, who realized that the tax revenues were needed to keep his budget viable. A recent analysis of medical and public health records in Russia found alcohol to be the cause of more than half of all Russian deaths between the ages of fifteen and fifty-four years.[6] According to the World Health Organization, one in five Russian men now die because of alcohol-related causes (compared to 6% of men globally).[7] To quote *West Side Story*, a large number of men in Russia might certainly say, "I got a social disease." Culture, not only biology, can clearly play a role in the genesis of alcoholic behavior. There is no more compelling measure of the consequences of a disease than the deaths it causes, and physicians will often define a disease in terms of what leads to mortality, as in high cholesterol leading to lipid-laden plaques in a cardiac artery. So we see in Russia that a *culture* of heavy drinking can define this outcome.

Another aspect of social causation is the style of drinking. Finland is a country where episodes of very heavy, "explosive" drinking are common, and these are often characterized by violent behavior. Finland and Sweden are countries adjacent to each other but culturally different. Both have high rates of alcohol consumption, but overall murder rates in Finland are more than twice that of Sweden. Finns commit murder while drunk almost twice as often as Swedes, and Finnish murders take place only a third as often during actual criminal activity, like robberies.[8] That is to say, Finns with alcohol problems are more likely to get very drunk, and when they do, they are likely to get violent in social situations. Violence, a potential pathology in defining alcoholism, can be said to be culturally determined in Finnish culture. Advice: Do not get into a fight with a drunk in Finland.

PERCEPTIONS OF ADDICTION

It is easy to say that alcoholism is a disease, as reflected in AA's First Step,[9] "We admitted that we are powerless over alcohol . . .," and then to validate it with patient accounts that bespeak its nature. Capturing the nature of the disease, however, reveals some very different ways of characterizing it. Each one has its own validity, and in a sense they are complementary. In other respects, they bespeak very different relationships at the nexus of mind, brain, culture, and behavior, let alone what each one suggests in terms of application to treatment.

We can consider each and all of them. A biological model of alcoholism as a disease has served as the basis for an investment among the medical research community in pharmacological solutions to the problem, such as medications that decrease alcohol craving. The biobehavioral conditioning model, alternatively, embodies an approach that has led to the application of cognitive-behavioral therapy to help people learn how alcohol triggers generate cravings that can lead to drinking. The psychoanalytic model looks at addiction in a different way, positing unconscious forces that can bring about relapse because of conflicts within each respective alcoholic person. Then there is a public health-oriented model, which extends the concept to less problematic levels of drinking, suggesting that there are various kinds of interventions that clinicians can apply, from a brief episode of counseling up to intensive intervention. Psychiatry presents an "official" view of diagnosis, but one which has evolved over time. I thought it useful to also include a popular view of alcoholism, as illustrated in motion pictures. In many respects, the common sense inherent in members of the lay public may lead to an understanding of alcoholism as good or valid as that of the experts.

We can begin here with the first of these conceptions.

The Biologic Model

This book is not a setting for spelling out the many complexities that have been developed under this rubric, but I think it is useful to begin with how they emerged, and where we now stand on them. One place to begin is the history of the "Narcotic Farm" in Lexington, Kentucky, operated by the U.S. Public Health Service as a hospital for addicted people. It was active as a research facility from the 1930s to the end of the 1960s. The farm was conceived as a setting where heroin addicts, primarily, could be hospitalized on the assumption that this retreat might eventually lead to some improvement in their illness. But the setting also became a major site for research into the nature of addiction, in terms of what happens with intoxication and withdrawal, and how these syndromes can be managed. "Lexington" included sophisticated researchers whose intention was to elaborate on what we could understand about addiction and its biology, in order to get a handle on what was seen as an intractable illness.

At the same time, researchers there and at some university medical centers were studying the nature of the alcohol withdrawal syndrome. This was the alcohol problem that was most preoccupying to doctors, because that is what they saw as so damaging in the hospitals. They did not have a very good idea about how to go about discouraging further drinking after a patient got over the acute phase.

By the early 1970s, there were enough advances in the addiction field to lead the National Institute of Mental Health to spin off two research institutes: the National Institute on Drug Abuse and the National Institute on Alcohol Abuse and Alcoholism. These were soon incorporated under the umbrella of the National Institutes of Health, which is strongly oriented toward biological treatments. This has set the tone for the support of research of a biological nature into addiction to alcohol and other drugs. Most recently, this area of research has addressed the physiology of addiction and changes in functions such as neurotransmission that characterize these illnesses. Much has been made of alcoholism and drug addiction as "brain diseases," and this has been vividly illustrated in metabolic studies of brain function, complemented by looking at changes that can be visualized with sophisticated brain imaging techniques.

These models for addiction start off with the observation of increased concentration of the neurotransmitter dopamine at the level of neuron synapses during drug intoxication. Chronic use can apparently lead to reduction in the dopamine receptors available in certain brain areas, which can persist for months after detoxification. This deficit is found to be associated with drug cravings, and can be tested by giving addicted subjects a choice of the drug or a cash award. It has been shown in these studies that addicted subjects are more likely to select a drug over the alternative of getting the monetary reward. The changes also are thought to alter the relationship between brain sites (in the prefrontal cortex) that regulate impulses and areas (in the limbic system) that are "rewarded" by drug use. The limbic system generates many behaviors that are instinctual in nature. We will discuss this further in the chapter on how AA "changes the brain."

The biologic model is clearly supported by research findings, but is primarily premised on observations made in addicted people during periods of actual drug use, or during the early stages of recovery after they were detoxified. It does not necessarily apply to the changes that may come about in long-term recovery, changes that may be related to why people cannot stop drinking or using drugs.

Because culture and peer influence clearly affect the likelihood of doing things that can lead to addiction, it has become more current now to add "in a social context" to the "brain disease" model, acknowledging that it is not all biologic. Nonetheless, the biological mechanism has served as the basis for research on a variety of agents that can modify the metabolic pathways associated with them. Some of these are helpful in alcoholism, but we certainly have a very long way to go before finding a silver bullet, if one even exists, for alcoholism, for cocaine, or for a large number of designer drugs now emerging.

Behavioral Conditioning

One of the leading researchers in the Lexington, Kentucky Narcotic Farm was Abraham Wikler, a psychiatrist who had studied the work of the Russian physiologist Ivan Pavlov, whose research on conditioned behavior has been highly influential. Wikler pondered over just what characteristics of a drug that could generate addiction and which could distinguish it from the many substances that can be imbided but never produce addictive behavior.[10] He came up with these characteristics: They produce a positive subjective feeling, and they generate a physiologic response associated with withdrawal symptoms of that very same agent.

Let me elaborate on this. Addictive drugs are said to be reinforcing, which is to say they produce an effect that may be obvious, as with alcohol or cocaine, or more subtle, as with nicotine. People—or laboratory mice for that matter—once they start taking such a drug "like" the response and feeling, and are inclined to continue taking more. This positive response can be most compelling, as in the case of Bill W, the cofounder of AA. He found that when he started drinking as a youth he felt a relief from distress and euphoria unlike any he had previously experienced.[11] But many a college student also can talk about the good feelings engendered by drinking. (Never mind the fact that after a night of drinking one can experience a hangover or remorse. This only comes later, and it does not offer a level of aversion that predominates over the first positive response experienced while drinking.)

The second characteristic of an addictive drug is that it can produce what Wikler called a counteradaptive response. That is to say, when the drug is imbibed, the body, through its innate response to this drug, attempts to restore equilibrium by responding in the opposite direction. This contrary response can be evident most clearly in the shakes that an alcoholic can experience the day after a binge, which is effectively the opposite of the sedative quality of the alcohol itself. Similarly, a binge on cocaine, an excitant, is followed by an emotional letdown, even depression.

This model posits that the counteradaptive response can be conditioned to be elicited by feelings, settings, or even people that regularly have been associated with the use of the drug. The conditioning takes place similar to the conditioning of Pavlov's dogs. In that case, Pavlov set up experiments with dogs so he could measure their salivation when offered food, while at the same time ringing a bell. If he did this enough times, the dog would salivate even if only the bell itself were rung. This salivating to the rings of the bell is called a conditioned reflex, as compared with an innate naturally reflexive response to food.

With regard to alcohol, if one regularly drank when feeling depressed, in time, feeling depressed could reflexively produce that conditioned counteradaptive response, which the chronic drinker experiences as alcohol craving. In fact, even before the craving is experienced, alcohol seeking behavior can take place by reflex. This alcohol seeking can be in the form of deciding to go to a bar, without even consciously knowing what triggered it. This model suggests that if the addicted person can become aware of the triggers that lead to episodes of drinking, he can be alerted to the vulnerability of relapse and thus can learn to recognize triggers and avoid future trouble. Alternatively, he may impulsively, it would seem suddenly, relapse to use. What AA and cognitive behavioral therapy do is help the addicted person recognize these triggers and avoid them or suppress a relapse-related response. This model was attractive to me when I first started out in the addiction field, especially when patients described the times they would relapse to drink. Along with the patient, I found that we could ferret out these triggers even if they had not been apparent to them initially.[12]

This conditioned reaction was dramatically evident in the case of heroin addicts who were free from drugs while in jail, and then released long after they had experienced any acute withdrawal symptoms. Some reported that upon arriving in their old neighborhood they developed acute withdrawal symptoms: The conditioned stimulus of the neighborhood setting, so frequently paired with drug taking in the years before they were jailed had precipitated the counteradaptive response. They experienced this response as withdrawal and craving, and this would sometimes lead to a relapse, much to their distress.

I saw this when I started interviewing addicted people. Street crime due to the heroin epidemic had been rampant. One could not park one's car overnight without risking the loss of its contents. Everyone knew that the "drug addicts" were responsible for this. For teaching purposes, I wanted to get at what the experience was like from the vantage point of an addicted person. I videotaped my interview with Eddie, who had been imprisoned for over two years for committing a robbery to feed his habit. He told me that he had relapsed shortly after returning to the old neighborhood from prison.

The interview was telling because Eddie seemed to have no idea why he impulsively shot up a heroin dose at that time. He said he had been pleased to be out of jail and abstinent, but had surprised himself because he had not wanted to return to heroin. But then,

> The decision that I reached was I'm gonna do this and that's it. I got money in my pocket. I put all my responsibility behind me, and went and satisfied myself.

With some prompting, I was able to get him to recall circumstances that he had long forgotten, such as a phone call to his old girlfriend. They had argued on the phone.

> So, you hang up the phone. At the moment you were hanging up, were you intending to get any drugs?
> Yes, for the first time now.
> You decided during the conversation?
> Yes. But I hadn't been thinking about it before.
> Do you recall what it was about the conversation, what triggered it at what point?
> It could have been her tone of voice. What she let out of her mouth. I don't exactly remember.
> Did you feel rejected or angry?
> Both. Rejected and that made me get angry.
> Then something clicked and the decision came to mind?
> Never stopped to give it no thought.
> You didn't say, Is this a bad idea?
> No, never stopped to give it any thought.

The old neighborhood and the shock of rejection precipitated an impulsive action. Both represented conditioned stimuli for drug taking: The setting and the rejection were enough to trigger the behavior. Opiates like heroin are hard to beat, even with therapy and AA or NA support. Medications like methadone can be used for replacing the opiate and blocking heroin craving.

The Psychoanalytic Model

One perspective based on psychoanalytic thinking was put forward by Leon Wurmser,[13] who, among other professional activities, had assumed responsibility for the treatment of addicted patients on a clinic unit. As an analyst, Wurmser dealt with the unconscious, and tried to ferret out processes that reflected intense, if inapparent, feelings. They would not necessarily be clear, either to the patient or to a harried clinician, but could nonetheless govern the behavior of an addicted person. He pointed out that such people could unwittingly act out of sheer self-destructiveness. As one patient noted, "I progress, and suddenly I have an urge to break out, to destroy everything I've built up, and then I'm completely down for a month and slowly build [self-esteem and social accomplishment] up again."

He wrote that a relapse behavior begins with an event characterized by sadness, letdown, or loneliness. This can be reality-based or imagined, but it results in a sudden plummeting of self-esteem, which Wurmser termed a "narcissistic crisis." Next comes an overwhelming feeling that cannot be articulated in words, an intense sense of rage, shame, or despair. He calls this an "affect regression," falling into an uncontrollable set of feelings due to a collapse of psychological defenses. This then yields to a sense of restlessness or craving. This can take place without the patient's conscious awareness or can be aborted before it actually takes place by reaching for a drink or a drug. One defense that this can bring about is that of denial, loss of recognition of the impulsive pressure. Wurmser avowed that the denial can be of psychotic or near-psychotic proportions.

All this may sound rather florid, but it should be pointed out that from a psychoanalytic perspective, deeply held feelings can lie beneath the surface of one's thinking in turbulent form and can be aborted by some impulsive act. Here is an example of this. In some large law firms, attorneys receive sizable bonuses at the end of each year based on points they are given by the firm's compensation committee, whose deliberations are typically cloaked in secrecy. One patient of mine who had been abstinent for some months was soon to get notice of the points assigned him. The notice came while he was sitting in his office, and it was for much less than he had felt fair or had expected. Without thinking, he rushed out of the office, went to a liquor store, bought a bottle of vodka, took it back and drank a good bit right out of the bottle. As he and I discussed after the fact, the mechanism of an aborted profound despair and, as Wurmser would put it, narcissistic injury was so compelling that he could only respond impulsively to the resulting reaction.

Lance Dodes, another psychoanalyst, gave me a similar explanation, and illustrated it with an alcoholic patient of his who had been standing on a street corner waiting for his wife who was doing some shopping.[14] He had dropped her off and had done some errands himself; they were supposed to meet at a certain time on the street corner. At the appointed time she did not show up. He waited and waited, and was unable to reach her. He became increasingly frustrated, saw a bar across the street, went in, and began to drink. At first he reported he had felt better after ordering the drink, but then following the experience back in time, he said that the truth of it was that he really started to feel better when he made the decision, while standing on the corner, to go get the drink. Along with the analyst, the patient concluded that he had felt totally helpless when he was standing on the corner. Dodes says that such relapses are due to a sense of utter powerlessness, and as such, powerlessness can underlie addictive behavior. In the analytic session, the two further figured out the relationship of such feelings to the patient's earlier life experiences. Dodes presumes that therapy can liberate a person from the compulsion to drink in this manner.

This psychoanalytic conception of the disease can be used in therapeutic sessions, not only by an analyst, but by other therapists as well, to begin to tease out the feelings that fuel the compulsion of addiction. The problem is that most busy clinicians do not have the time that a psychoanalyst may have to deploy in examining such conflicts. Indeed, such examinations in the view of many may be of insufficient value in terminating a pattern of addictive behavior in most cases.

A model like this may allow addiction to remain defined as a nondisease, and seeming far removed from physical dysfunction and disability. Nonetheless, many psychoanalysts are, in fact, physicians, psychiatrists who treat the body as well as the mind, at least by their prior training. They may also prescribe medications, but look to mental mechanisms when trying to understand their patients.

A Psychiatric Perspective

For a long time, psychiatry has grappled with how to define addiction and how to organize a related model of treatment. Benjamin Rush was a physician and a signatory to the Declaration of Independence; his image has been emblazoned on the logo of the American Psychiatric Association. Rush was attentive to the problems of alcohol, because his father suffered from alcoholism. His broader approach to this issue emerged in relation to the Continental Army. Drunkenness was a problem among soldiers, and General George Washington was also aware of the problem. Rush condemned the soldiers' access to distilled spirits.

Psychiatry's understanding of the issue of addiction as a disease is not graven in stone. I have been in a good position to see some of this evolution over the last decades, having served as President of the American Academy of Addiction Psychiatry and, for twenty years, as a member of the Addiction Council of the American Psychiatric Association. When I was a resident in psychiatry, the faculty at my medical school focused on unconscious motivation and on the role of affect (feelings) governing a person's life. It was thought that this could lead to unraveling the mystery of dysfunctional behavior in a lengthy series of therapy sessions. I remember visiting the Maudsley Hospital in London as a medical student. It was the mecca of academic psychiatry in Great Britain then, as it is now. I encountered a different brand of psychiatry there; case conferences revolved around attempts to focus diagnosis on the possibility of palpable brain damage, such as subdural hematomas. It seemed a bit strange, but it did herald a change coming about in psychiatry. A few years later I visited a friend and colleague at Washington University in St. Louis, a leading setting for the rejection of psychoanalysis as a model for treatment, and spoke with the residents there. They were concerned for their patients and quite pragmatic in helping them out, but for them consideration of unconscious motives was in no way part of their language.

The American Psychiatric Association's *Diagnostic and Statistical Manual of Mental Illness II* of 1968[15] had listed addiction as a personality disorder and described it in narrative form, but a change was going to emerge in the APA's next lexicon. The DSM III, released in 1980,[16] conformed to a model developed in the early 1970s under the intellectual leadership of psychiatrist George Winokur, who felt that analysts just dealt with the "problems of daily living," rather than mental illness. Psychoanalysis was falling into disrepute in academic psychiatry, and the APA was now attempting to create a system for diagnosis that would be "objective" and based on observation.

The new diagnostic manual reflected the movement away from lending weight to understanding the subjective experiences of people. Psychiatric diagnosis was now intended to make assessments based on manifest symptoms as much as possible, rather than reflecting on the painful or personally meaningful experiences in patients' lives. Because of this, each of the diagnoses had a list of demonstrable symptoms associated with it. If the number of symptoms a patient had added up properly, this now made for a diagnosis.

With regard to alcohol and other drugs, the attempt also was made to remove negative prejudicial connotations. Thus, a person was diagnosed as someone with "alcohol dependence" rather than being an "alcoholic." In both the *DSM III* and the 1994 *DSM IV*,[17] symptoms of alcohol withdrawal (like the morning-after shakes) and tolerance (needing to drink more to get the same effect) were included as options for making a diagnosis. If one had three or more symptoms of the nine listed, one could now be diagnosed as having the illness of alcohol dependence. But, truth to tell, even these items could reflect the subjective view of the clinician. For example, how bad does a "recurrent social or interpersonal problem" have to be before being listed for a given person as a diagnostic symptom? Or now, in the *DSM V*[18] of 2013, how badly does one have to crave alcohol (a new addition to the diagnostic list) in order to qualify for "craving?"

Let's consider the *DSM V*, and why "craving" now has been added to the list of criteria. It is not because craving was not an issue for the alcoholic before the manual's revision. It did, however, reflect the view of the head of the committee that framed the new criteria. He had been instrumental in the development of newly emerging anticraving drugs, and earnestly intent on seeing them used more widely, so it seemed like craving should find a place in the diagnosis of alcoholism. (Admittedly, this is my opinion, and, importantly, none of the committee members had a financial stake in any of these emerging anticraving drugs.)

Before the *DSM V*, there was an option of diagnosing "alcohol abuse." It was designated for problem drinkers who were not severely compromised. The distinction between abuse and dependence was useful in the opinion of many psychiatrists because it could denote a syndrome that was more of a reaction to circumstances, effectively bad behaviors when one drank. This way one could distinguish someone who just got into trouble with occasional drinking, such as having an argument with her spouse about getting drunk at parties, and maybe even driving home while still under the influence. It differed from the compromised skid row alcoholic or the person who could just not stop drinking.

One interesting upshot of these transitions is that this approach somehow muddies the water regarding the "disease concept" of alcoholism, given that it now consists of eleven symptoms, which when tallied up, extend from the mild level of problem "alcoholic disorder" with two to three symptoms to the more severely compromised person, with six or more. It becomes harder to conceptualize the problem as a disease, however, when it ranges from a mild disorder of adaptation to what we think of as more severe. This somewhat complex system makes it harder to decide when to tell a patient that she or he "would do well to go to AA." The old distinction between alcohol abuse and dependence offered a clearer distinction of the latter category, which connoted addiction. It would be easier to handle a diagnosis that clearly suggests a particular course of treatment.

And I see this in clinical practice. Although the DSM is used for diagnosis in research, it is still a lexicon to help clinicians embark on treating their patients. When a clinician wants a patient to begin a course of treatment that involves getting over the hurdle of resistance and going to an AA meeting, it is good to have something clear and explicit to base it on—alcoholic or not—rather than a series of symptoms: mild, moderate, or severe. This latter approach now adopted, in terms of talking to the patient, gives a doctor a less clear demarcation for telling the patient he or she must take an action and actually expose him- or herself to the idea of going to AA.

A Public Health Perspective

Alcohol problems are remarkably costly to our society. According to the U.S. Centers for Disease Control, they kill 79,000 Americans each year.[19] In addition, the overall economic burden placed on our country by these disorders is $230 billion by one accounting. The cost of treatment constitutes only 11% of this; the majority of the overall burden (72%) comes from lost productivity,[20] a burden that is often not appreciated.

Because of figures like this, the U.S. federal government has in recent decades taken an active role in combating this disease, with major investments in research, treatment, and innovative program development. One approach has been to look broadly at the nature of alcohol's impact on people. Based on national surveys, federal reports construct a triangle, representing 100% of the population. It looks like the food triangle of what one should eat, with layers of various sizes. The lowest 74% have no substantial problem with alcohol at all. Moving up toward the top, 23% do not have alcohol dependence, but they do binge or use alcohol excessively. Only a small portion, namely 3.3%, are considered alcohol dependent. What this means, in effect, is that for every American adult who is alcoholic, as we have labeled the disease, more than some six others are not dependent, but have had material problems with their drinking. This larger group is considered "at risk." They may have fewer severe alcohol-related problems, such as accidents or problematic social behavior, but they are not "addicted" to alcohol, so to speak. This larger group is represented by some of the people who appear at medical trauma centers, where almost half of the patients come in with positive blood alcohol levels.

It is thought that this larger population, when they appear for medical treatment in either emergency room settings or doctors' offices, should undergo screening for alcohol problems, followed by a brief interaction with advice from the caregiver, one that is thought to lead to a decrease in problem drinking, and ultimately a decrease in healthcare costs. One might question, though, whether these latter folks fit into the "disease" of alcoholism that we have been talking about, or for that matter, whether the focus of this approach on these alcohol problems might in some way detract from attending to people who are more severely diseased.

Nonetheless, the U.S. federal government has focused considerable attention on the problems such people represent.

With all this in mind, government agencies have come to promote an approach called screening and brief intervention. Here is how they suggest the treating person, be it a doctor or nurse, in the outpatient office, the emergency room, or the hospital, go about this process. First, the patient is given feedback as to what specific issue, such as their score on a screening questionnaire or blood alcohol level, has raised the issue for discussion. Then in a motivational way, the clinician should, with the patient, try to understand the nature of the drinking in question. For example, if they are injured and in the emergency room, they might discuss how drinking might have played a role in the injury, and they might be asked if they thought it would be useful to change their drinking habits. The idea is to do this in a collaborative way rather than in a confrontational fashion. Finally, based on this arrived-at mutuality, the patient can be given advice, along with some discussion about what the clinician thinks would be a reasonable approach to undertake. This might be cutting back on drinking or, in a more problematic situation, even quitting drinking altogether. In the latter case, a referral for treatment would be appropriate. The idea here is to be supportive and nonjudgmental.

This idea sounds good, and might, in fact, be a way to address the problem of drinking overall. What emerged from well-controlled research,[21] however, was that while there was indeed some benefit from the screening and brief intervention process in primary care settings for the at-risk population, for patients with alcohol addiction, the 3.3% on top of the triangle, no benefit was found. This was clearly true in the hospital setting, where the most compromised alcoholics are found. And the approach, for that matter, has not been demonstrated to be effective for drug problems either.

This whole conception harkens back to findings such as those reported by George Vaillant[22] over thirty years ago, when he carried out extensive studies on members of a Boston community who had alcohol problems. He noted a series of sixteen symptoms for interviewees, ones that they might have relative to alcohol problems, and found that those who responded positively to fewer than half of them had varying degrees of potentially engaging in social drinking without being symptomatic. Of those with more than half the symptoms, however, none had been able to return to a symptom-free state without becoming totally abstinent. It is this latter group who are the best candidates for AA.

Defined in the Movies

One interesting thing about alcoholism is that its portrayal in the public mind and the media may do the best job of capturing its nature as a gravely serious disease, and for this we can actually turn to feature films to develop a lexicon of its characteristics.

The Lost Weekend (1945) won the Oscar for Best Picture in its year. It is a virtual catalog of the defining aspects of alcoholism and its destructive nature. Ray Milland plays Don, a failed author and an alcoholic. At best, he is refined; at worst, he is desperate. He relapses to drinking after a period of sobriety when he is overcome by anxiety upon overhearing his potential in-laws discussing his character flaws. He repeatedly rejects offers of help from his girlfriend—illustrating the denial of illness and the tenacious unwillingness of the alcoholic, even in the throes of illness, to acknowledge a need for help. His drinking is punctuated by the symptom of hiding liquor bottles to protect his access, by a rope outside his window and then in an overhead light fixture. Further vulnerability to triggers for drinking is revealed when Don witnesses the drinking song at an operatic performance of "La Traviata" and rushes off to have a drink from a flask in his coat pocket. A fall while drunk results in his being knocked unconscious. All this devolves into hallucinatory experiences when he comes to the point of being in delirium tremens (DTs), that is, life-threatening withdrawal. (By the way, he is taken to a hospital that is clearly the old Bellevue building, famous for its detox ward, where I set up our alcoholism clinic years later.) At the end of the film, Don chooses a try at recovery when he drops a cigarette into a whiskey glass rather than taking a drink. You could lay out criteria for a diagnosis for the disease from this movie alone: denial of illness, resisting help, relapse on encountering an alcohol trigger, hiding one's drinking, medical consequences.

Leaving Las Vegas (1995) is the tragic tale of a man, played by Nicholas Cage, who had lost everything to alcohol: his job, his family, and his friends. The despair of the alcoholic is palpable in its presentation in this film, and one can see self-hatred in this man's face and in his every word. He now goes to Las Vegas to drink himself to death. While driving drunk down the Strip, he almost hits a woman in the crosswalk. He then checks into a sleazy hotel, where he solicits Sera, a prostitute, and starts a relationship with her. She later pleads with him to see a doctor and get help. His angry response, reflecting the alcoholic's defensiveness when confronted, is to bring another prostitute to her house, resulting in her kicking him out. He continues to drink heavily, never eating, and in time he and Sera make up and have sex. As Sera sleeps, he dies with her in his arms. The film captures what AA labels as a disease of despair, which unresolved, can lead to death. In doing this, it conveys the potentially terminal nature of the illness more clearly than do our professionally generated definitions.

The fact that alcohol is not only a disease of the individual but also one of the family is portrayed in the next two films. *Come Back Little Sheba* (1952) starring Burt Lancaster as Doc, illustrates how alcoholism can develop after a tragic turn in life. Doc's wife lost the capacity to bear children after the death of their first child, and he then started drinking heavily. He is now an abstinent AA member, but seems to be rigidly self-controlling at all times. As the movie progresses, he falls prey to jealous anger over the relationship of their attractive co-ed tenant with a boyfriend. He takes the whiskey bottle he kept at home as lingering evidence of his sobriety, gets drunk, falls into the kind of venomous rage that alcohol can drive one to, and attacks his wife with a knife. Fortunately, she is able to summon his fellow AA members who take him to a hospital. In the end, he and his wife reconcile. The film gives an example of the erratic moods and gravely serious violence that can accompany the disease.

Alcoholics can certainly compromise their kids as Meg Ryan, playing Alice, does in the film, *When a Man Loves a Woman* (1994). When drunk, she seems to care little about anything but drinking. She neglects her children, slaps her eldest daughter, and then falls down, breaking through a shower door. In a panic, the daughter summons her father to fly home from another city from his work as a pilot. Alice ends up in rehab, and she and her husband separate, leaving him responsible for the kids and now attending Al Anon meetings. In the end, Alice establishes herself in sobriety, and resumes the role of caretaker for the children. When she tells her story at an AA meeting after 180 days' sobriety, her husband reappears and they embrace. This is a benign outcome, where rehab is given a positive review and Al Anon provides the husband with a constructive view of the needs of his wife. In the film, we witness alcoholism as a disease where one can lose the capacity to love, and then see remission as a benign possibility in the face of the continued caring between a couple.

But more tragedy: James Mason plays a matinee idol whose career is in decline in *A Star is Born* (1954). He promotes an opening for a young woman (Judy Garland) who tries to save him during her own ascent to stardom, but he cannot avoid making a fool of himself on stage while drunk. Judy Garland lovingly does all she can do to cover up for him, even telling an audience that his barging on the stage is part of a theatrical act. Ultimately, he goes off for a swim to drown himself in the ocean. Humiliation and suicide are outcomes for some alcoholics, and completed suicides are most often associated with alcoholism.

Many talented writers over the last century have suffered from alcoholism, and they themselves yield a catalog of symptoms that define the disease. James Joyce famously binged and fought in bars. Ernest Hemingway committed suicide. Tennessee Williams, Truman Capote, and William Faulkner managed to survive their drinking while committed to their writing. Dylan Thomas, Jack Kerouac, and F. Scott Fitzgerald did not. John Cheever survived after rehab and AA.

The poet Charles Bukowski, portrayed by Mickey Rourke in the film *Barfly* (1987), spent his writing life drinking heavily. The penchant of some alcoholics for violence and despoiling their career opportunities while drunk is captured most vividly in a failed encounter with a literary sponsor who wants to support him in his work. Bukowski never seeks redemption, and as he wrote in one of his poems, "when you drank the world was still out there, but for the moment it didn't have you by the throat." And indeed, as portrayed in the film, Bukowski was able to forget that his drinking, rather than "the world," is what had him by the throat.

So alcoholism can be clearly and vividly portrayed on film, rather than in the variety of scientifically grounded research endeavors. Film can capture it in its full pathology, defining the true and grave disease as we know it. Here are the symptoms we saw from which alcoholism could be diagnosed, based on these movies alone: denial, hiding liquor bottles, environmental and emotional triggers, potential DTs with hallucinations, despair, interpersonal conflict, unstable mood and rage when drinking, neglect of family responsibilities, potential suicide, and disrupted career and work life. And this is just from these six films. The popular media may give us a better picture of the disease then do the "experts."

Denial

The cliché that "denial" is not just a river in Egypt is not just a humorous turn of phrase. It points to the barrier to recovery that, in practice, is what makes it hardest to move on to recovery from addiction. It is key to why AA needs to effect a transformation in the addicted person's understanding of himself. This involves taking people embedded in a falsity of how they experience the way they have been leading their lives and somehow turning this around. We need to consider this further.

The alcoholic characters in the movies just described clearly balked at the help offered them and responded angrily to those who most cared for their well-being. Even with the disease these folks have, they cannot acknowledge their need to stay away from the bottle. This is because of denial, the characteristic of alcoholism that is so commonly a part of this affliction. It is a term embedded in AA members' parlance, and is a key to the difficulties that doctors like me have to overcome in treating addicted people. However important it actually is, it is not specified as a symptom among the psychiatric diagnostic criteria for the disease, perhaps because it is an unconsciously mediated mental mechanism. Researchers who had originally formulated the criteria were not comfortable with terms that reflected unconscious processes the likes of which Freudian psychology employs. Nonetheless, we need to look further at this consistently observed symptom and try to understand it.

A classic example of denial is regularly encountered in hospital settings, when an alcoholic patient in grave medical condition is suffering from its life-threatening consequences, such as liver failure due to cirrhosis or multiple organ failure due to pancreatitis. Most all physicians during their training have encountered "impossible" patients like these who, when asked how much they have been drinking, answer to the effect of "hardly at all" or "I've been staying away from the stuff recently." It is hard to understand how the patient can believe what he is saying, but he apparently does seem to think that he is answering honestly.

Other examples of denial are less flagrant. A patient of mine, long in recovery, and correctly desirous of understanding what his drinking had cost his family, brought his adult son into a session one time when the young man was visiting from out of state. When I asked the son about some of the consequences of his father's drinking, he told of episodes when he and a girlfriend were quite innocently in a room by themselves. Dad would shout angrily, then run upstairs, and pound on his door. Not all of these events took place when dad was drunk enough to be in a blackout. The patient himself was dismayed to find out about these outbursts, and was surprised and ashamed to hear of his behavior.

One question about initiating a positive course of treatment for an alcoholic is how to undermine such denial, given that it is important for patients to be aware of the actual consequences of their drinking in order to be motivated to change. In AA, this is promoted by requiring speakers on the podium who recount their drinking experiences ("qualify") to begin by saying "I'm ___, and I'm an alcoholic," so that they cannot avoid the reality of their alcoholism.

When I first see alcoholic patients in the consulting room, I prefer to do so with a family member joining in so that a more valid recounting of the problem will come out in the session, rather than it being clouded by a patient's denial. I have the family member fill in details of the story of drinking-related behaviors to illuminate the issue as the session progresses. More compelling details always emerge, like when the patient fell down drunk at a family wedding; when people at the office would call up and ask why he was not in that day; when their five-year-old son would erupt in tears when Dad was screaming during a drinking bout.

Denial, as a psychologically determined maneuver, was described by Sigmund Freud and, in more detail, by his daughter Anna Freud in her classic work, *The Ego and the Mechanisms of Defense*.[23] She wrote how unconsciously generated, threatening feelings can be diverted in the mind in a variety of ways to avoid the experience of conscious distress. One such mechanism is suppression, whereby a person actively attempts to do away with, to ignore, the offending thoughts. An alcoholic may do this as a prelude to lying about alcohol. More pathologically, however, because it reflects a loss of contact with reality, unconscious processes may bury the offending thoughts without any awareness on the part of the person herself, so that she does not actively deal with the associated distress. It is this process that takes place in the examples of denial I just described.

Are there findings from recent brain research that can shed light on the process of denial? In fact, there are problems in undertaking this that are hard to overcome. The most confounding aspect of doing such research on alcoholic denial is that people in denial, like those mentioned above, are not consistently available for evaluation by techniques such as MRI scanning. Neither are their examples of denial consistent enough among them respectively to allow comparisons to be readily made between such subjects.

But it would be useful to draw some inferences from recent studies that can shed light on this process, as well as the psychodynamic interpretations of the denial of the illness. We can put it this way: The denying alcoholic seems to ignore past behaviors and problems, thereby effectively avoiding the conscious discomfort of looking at the consequences of his acts. Do we have any idea what processes in the brain are associated with this?

There has been a good deal of brain scanning research in recent years on the process of lying. Results of this have even shown up in the courts, where imaging has been entered as evidence, but is typically questioned in terms of its evidentiary value. Martha Farah and her colleagues[24] illustrated the state of this work in their review of a study in which one group of subjects was asked to commit a simulated crime, while a second group was not asked. Here is how this worked[25]: Subjects were taken to a specific room and told to "steal" a watch or ring that had been placed in a specific drawer, and were then told to deny doing this. Other subjects were not told to "steal" these items. Both groups were instructed to deny that they had done so. The ones who were "lying" (who had actually done the stealing) were detected with accuracy by fMRI. So far so good. The only problem was that many of the ones who had not committed the crime, and were telling the truth, had the fMRI pattern of "lying" as well. That is to say, they were false positives. So we do see some progress in imaging the process of lie detection, but it is clearly fallible.

There also has been a significant body of research on how emotionally charged events are remembered differently than more neutrally experienced ones. This is can be done by showing people relevant words, film clips, or stories that include a destructive or sexual connotation. These experiences, when retrieved from memory, are associated with greater activation of limbic structures, parts of the human brain that mediate instinctually based activation (the amygdala in particular).[26] Such studies may open the door to consideration of how a denying person, having long suppressed feelings associated with drinking, might show a different pattern of activation tied in with conscious denial of experiences related to their drinking.

Forgetting, in fact, may be shown on imaging to have an adaptive function in reducing the demands on brain centers associated with actively controlling problematic memories. In studies where conflicting memories are forgotten, it has been found that there is a reduction in the need to suppress the experience of the conflict (as measured in the anterior cingulate cortex) along with decreased activation in the location where memory suppression takes place (in the prefrontal cortex).[27] That is to say, when a person is under stress, forgetting can relieve the brain areas that suppress certain memories.

How does this play out for someone who has been lying more habitually? One study on criminal offenders diagnosed with an antisocial personality disorder may shed light on this.[28] People with this disorder often lie without even thinking about it. When the offenders were given a psychometric test that measured how deceptive they were, those who showed up as most deceptive on the test were deemed the best deceivers. All the offenders studied were told to choose three pictures out of the ones presented to them and then later lie and say they had picked ones they really had not picked. In offenders who had been found to be the best deceivers, the brain centers that exercise active control over suppression showed less activation during the "lying" than they showed in the offenders who were not good deceivers. That is to say, intuitive, automatic deception, in someone who is used to it does not need to summon up brain centers responsible for actively suppressing the act of deception. This may be what happens in an alcoholic who has been in denial for long enough to give false reports about his drinking without even thinking about it.

In time, such research may provide us with a bridge between the psychodynamic model of denial and the physiology that underlies it. It may help us to understand better how an addicted person's falsification can become habituated by repeatedly deceiving him or herself and thus relieving the stress of guilt and shame over not being able to control the drinking or drug use. In the case of the alcoholic, the stress is one of facing a depressing reality, as stated in the First Step of AA, "powerlessness over alcohol."

CHAPTER 3

How I Got Involved

Because Alcoholics Anonymous is controversial in many ways, you, the reader, would do well to see how I have tried to be objective in pursuing this task, and make a judgment on your own about the various aspects of the movement and how they are described here. You should know that I have been a clinician treating addicted people; an acquaintance of a good number of AA members, although not a member myself; a researcher of social movements and of AA itself; and supportive of the fellowship's more effective use in helping addicted people.

One limitation in achieving an objective assessment of AA is that no researcher has been given access to the movement itself by the fellowship's General Service Office. As we have said, AA zealously protects the anonymity of its members. It does not keep lists of who they are and how they have progressed, and it does not collaborate with any outside organizations or academic institutions. Most of the research that had been done has looked at how people fare in a follow-up after they leave professionally run treatment programs, since some treatment programs do cooperate with researchers. But the people who are studied there do not represent the many who encounter AA on their own, who are referred by a doctor in private practice, or for that matter, who are referred by a distraught friend who wants to be of help. The people who have been followed up after treatment—and for a limited time at that— also do not include those who drop out and then return, and who have then stayed on with long-term ties to the fellowship. I have done studies myself within these constraints. Because of this, a comprehensive assessment inevitably has to include a fair-minded attempt to draw on the respective experiences of many members. I have tried to do this as well.

After doing research related to AA, I was chairing committees on Twelve Step recovery for the two American medical addiction societies. Having previously served as president of both of the Societies, I was accorded some latitude on this. It was a problem that so many of my colleagues in these societies had a limited understanding of Twelve Step programs and were not making optimal use of them, even though Twelve Step meetings could be so easily accessed by their patients. And these doctors were the supposed experts in addiction treatment, some four thousand of them in all. What about the other hundreds of thousands of health professionals not designated as expert, but encountering addicted patients nonetheless?

Our two committees conducted workshops where mock AA meetings were held for the Society attendees, followed by a discussion of the experience. These were informative because of the very personal nature of what the members in these simulated meetings had to say. What seemed necessary, though, was to provide data-based research in a manner that could lend credence to the utility of AA for the medical community. The medical field has (wisely) become oriented to "evidence-based" treatments, rather than ones derived from informed but potentially biased clinical experience. This meant that quantitatively framed studies with experimental controls were those that could be presented to doctors with an expectation of credibility. Only such research would carry the weight necessary to validate any modality for use in medical care.

FIELD STUDIES

So I hoped to orient the research I was doing to demonstrate the nature and relative effectiveness of the Twelve Step model to fellow physicians, but I needed support to pay staff for this. Data had to come from Twelve Step members themselves, but this could only be carried out as the opportunity might arise, because AA would not do this under contract with a university. Because it could not be scheduled or contracted long in advance, as federal research agencies like the National Institutes of Health would want, it would be hard to engage the government in this.

It turned out that officers of the John Templeton Foundation, familiar with the research I had done on the cultic religious youth movements some years before, as well as some studies on spirituality in AA, invited me to submit an application for support that could address a moving target like this under the rubric of spirituality in health promotion.

Admittedly, I had applied for this funding before being clear on how this entry into the Twelve Step universe could be assured, so I turned to

Bill C, a local AA officer who had been participating in our medical training on addiction. Were there any means of working out such a project? We devoted a good deal of time to discussing this with Daniel S, chairman of the local AA Committee on Professional Cooperation (CPC). Most of its members were positively disposed, realizing the value of such research, but AA moves very slowly, and does not undertake anything that is not achieved by full consensus. Because of this, in the end, old-time members on the CPC who voiced their reservations stymied any possibility of work with their AA committee on such a project. Bill and Daniel were remorseful; they had felt that this effort could ultimately provide a valuable contribution to doctors getting better engaged with AA.

By a fortunate coincidence, the upcoming International Conference of Young People in AA (YPAA) was to be held that year in New York at the massive forty-nine-story Marriott Marquis Hotel in Times Square. Bill and Daniel arranged for me to present the option of carrying out a research project there to members of the conference organizing committee. YPAA is constituted of AA members, but is not formally a part of the AA structure. This meant that they were at liberty to affiliate as they chose, and could agree to let someone outside the group do a study on their members.

When the day came to meet with the committee, Bill and I arrived at the Manhattan Veterans' Hospital and were informed by the security guard that there was no Young People's meeting there. Bill, however, knew where the meeting was to be held (Was its presence sanctioned?), and we went up to the eighteenth floor. We entered a large room with some forty people, on average younger than thirty, sitting around a very large conference table. Bill introduced me as a credible figure whose research could advance doctors' understanding of Twelve Step recovery, and I outlined an option that we could undertake at the time of the conference.

The way the committee members conducted their work was quite telling of the ability of AA to move young adults from severe disruption in their lives to competent function. I was impressed by the high degree of organization that these YPAA members had achieved. After all, these were folks who some time before had become addicted and severely compromised, and from an early age at that. Parliamentary procedure was followed, subcommittee reports were given, and a congenial, but business-like atmosphere persisted over the hour that Bill and I were there prior to giving our presentation. The reception was more positive than at the AA Committee on Professional Cooperation, in part because members of the group were younger and more open to the idea of research. Objections raised by some members were resolved by others on the planning committee.

My staff and I were given an opportunity to set up two tables at the planned conference near the registration area. Over the course of the conference, there was an opportunity to meet some remarkable young people whose tales of addiction were quite compelling, but who had now achieved a stable adaptation in work or school. People were helpful to us, and the organizing committee had even placed a notice in their conference program telling participants of our undertaking. It was specified, though, that this was not a function of the AA group itself, and attendees were invited to participate only if they chose to do so. My team and I selected 358 attendees at random to fill out a lengthy and carefully framed computer-scored survey instrument. Later, we were able to tabulate and ultimately publish our results in a peer-reviewed medical journal.[1] I also was able to present this material to some large medical audiences at conferences, with the ultimate goal of demonstrating the viability of the Twelve Step format even for teenagers and young adults.

ADDICTED PHYSICIANS

We were able to carry out further research on physicians in addiction recovery after a visit paid me by one doctor from upstate New York. He had presented some of my studies on spirituality and AA to the program committee of the annual meeting of International Doctors in AA, and this had met their expectation for empirical evidence on this aspect of the AA experience. The committee then let him focus on spirituality for their continuing medical education program. When I asked him if the attendees in his educational series would be willing to participate in our study about their own recovery, he was more than willing to help. With his cooperation and with the participation of a group of his colleagues, we were able to survey 324 attendees in two studies over the course of the doctors' annual conferences.[2]

When I asked the doctor from upstate New York whether he could speak with our fellows in training about his own experience with addiction, he did so. His story was remarkable with regard to his continuing abuse of alcohol and cocaine. During his initial monitoring by the New York State Medical Society's program for addicted physicians, he had been able to falsify his urine toxicologies to indicate abstinence. Now, at this point in his story, he could only express a degree of bemusement that he had successfully faked his initial course of treatment. He eventually did come around to realizing, admittedly under pressure from colleagues, that he had to embark seriously on the legitimate course of recovery he had now been carefully following for some years.

NARCOTICS ANONYMOUS

A most compelling example of Twelve Step recovery came from a group of veterans who were brought together by the Narcotics Anonymous (NA) central office after we had carried out an initial study on that fellowship. NA is a worldwide Twelve Step fellowship open to addicts of all drugs of abuse.

The initial idea of our working together came about at a conference of the International Society of Addiction Medicine. One person there was the president of a related organization, and was himself a physician in recovery. He had advanced from being a heroin addict sleeping in a bus terminal to attending medical school at Columbia University and then to a residency at John Hopkins—a truly remarkable story. He introduced me to NA representatives at the conference and said I was someone whom they could trust and with whom they could work. He was quite a charismatic fellow, and his introduction gave me entrée into their universe. This validation from someone in recovery, who also had achieved a leadership position in the medical field, was key to their agreeing to collaborate.

NA had emerged over a decade or two after AA was established, out of the need for heroin addicts to find a place where they could use the Twelve Steps to bolster their recovery; today it draws on people addicted to a diversity of drugs. Unlike AA, it is organized with an element of management from its central office, located in a suburb of Los Angeles. The public relations folks there had been able to engage local NA groups from four different states to participate in our study. Our results showed that the Twelve Step formula, with an attendant commitment to abstinence from drugs, applied well in that fellowship setting.[3,4]

Following this study, we discussed the possibility of looking into how NA helped addicted veterans. This was at a time when the Veterans Administration system was overburdened with many soldiers returning from the Middle East, many of whom had fallen prey to substance abuse and were in dire need of help. At first, the staff at the NA headquarters did not know how, from among their many groups, they could access the necessary number of veterans for us to evaluate, but they did agree to set up the focus group in New York to give us a better understanding of how NA helped veterans achieve recovery. The stories told at the focus group were most compelling. Most were Vietnam vets who served at a time when heroin use was rampant among the troops, and when returning soldiers were hardly told, "Thank you for your service," as those who served in Afghanistan and Iraq would later be told. They came home alienated because of their post-traumatic battle scars, their addictions, and Americans' distaste for the Vietnam War effort.

What they said in our focus group made clear how a community of shared belief had given them a new lease on life. The NA public relations representative and I were quite taken by their compelling stories. We realized that the role of recovery in the lives of these previously dejected people was a subject meriting attention, and it would be useful to get a compelling hearing for making best use of NA for veterans. It seemed like an excellent opportunity by which the medical community in the VA system could become aware of the value of this Twelve Step option, if based on an empirical study.

The NA central office reached out to groups of theirs around the country that had veterans among them, and I was able to apply our survey format to the particulars of military service, its emotional consequences, and symptoms of post-traumatic stress disorder. The resulting publication[5] demonstrated the way NA membership had successfully addressed the effects of combat and injury. This was particularly salient, because over half the veterans we surveyed reported that they had experienced symptoms associated with post-traumatic stress disorder. It reflected a way of addressing PTSD not even mentioned when members of the academic community reviewed the options available for treatment [6] of this major post-war problem.

HOW DOES ONE STUDY AA?

Before a book proposal is considered for publication by Oxford University Press, it is anonymously reviewed by scholars in the field. The proposal for this book was favorably reviewed, but one of the reviewers said that she or he was tired of hearing people's stories of recovery, and hoped that the book would focus on hard data. I think this epitomizes the distinction between what we learn from statistics culled across groups of people, and what actually happens to given individuals.

Let me make this more specific. The statistics that we get in the research literature are important and are understood to be "objective," but they do not capture the experience of what a given treatment does for a given individual. Here is an example of one such study, on the longest follow-up by far on alcoholics ever done, over sixteen years. It reflects a remarkable job by Rudolph Moos and Bernice Moos from Stanford University, who evaluated 461 alcoholic people who had made contact with the local alcohol treatment system. A key finding about AA emerged from this effort:[7]

> An initial episode of professional treatment may have a beneficial influence on alcohol-related functioning; however, continued participation in a community-based self-help program, such as AA, appears to be a more important determinant of long-term outcomes.

This they derived from careful reporting and data analysis. And it is very useful in validating the utility of AA in promoting alcohol recovery.

This kind of research can be termed positivist in nature, reflecting a concept developed by a nineteenth-century French father of sociology, August Comte. He wrote that an understanding of society needed to be premised on observable, and ideally measurable, phenomena.[8] But what this does not do is provide a sense of what experiences are like for given individuals who differ greatly among themselves, or of what their experiences mean to any of them. I will discuss some telling studies in this book, positivist in character, but will also, despite the reviewer's complaint, include a lot of experiences told in the words of addicted people themselves. This relates to a branch of research carried out by storytelling, based on a perspective—as the psychologist Jerome Bruner would have it—that is valid for scientific inquiry.[9]

To sum up, we embark here on a journey whose purpose is to understand "what AA is," and I try here to capture both the human side of this experience as well as to provide an objective look at what the fellowship is like.

PART II

The Alcoholics Anonymous Experience

CHAPTER 4

Engagement

Most people approach AA reluctantly. Here is how one woman described her experience after her therapist had told her she ought to go to a meeting:

> I decided to go so I could tell him about it because that was what he wanted to hear. I drove over to the church where it was held and sat outside in the parking lot. Then I drove around several times before I could get up the courage to walk into the building. I didn't like the idea that there were other people coming out. It was embarrassing. I didn't realize that they were alcoholics who had just come out of a first meeting. I didn't want to go past them. I just wanted them to go away so I could sneak into the meeting and see what I had to hear. I sucked up the courage and walked into that meeting room and stood by the door so I could escape.

An organized group that is designed to convey a new identity to its members, and then expecting them to behave accordingly, has to have a way of drawing them in. For fraternities, it is pledging and hazing; for the Army, it is recruitment and basic training; for the medical profession, it is cramming in specialized knowledge, followed by an arduous internship. AA presents a particular kind of induction, too. It has to get recruits to "turn [their] will and lives over to the care of God *as we understand Him*" (Third Step). And it has to get them to willingly give up an agent to which they are addicted. That is a lot to accomplish, and a lot for us to consider here.

In trying to understand how AA does this, I had found that studying the way people become members of zealous religiously oriented movements sheds light on the process. Here is how this came about. I was beginning to learn about AA as a junior faculty member treating addicted people. A Career Award offered time to study how AA could be used in treatment, but it also gave me time to do related research. As it happened, in the 1970s I got a chance to study some new religious youth movements that had a profound effect on their members. Their recruits forsook their family ties and religious backgrounds and became committed to leaders whose ideologies changed their outlook on life. The movements were often called cults, but they can suggest some broad outlines of how AA achieves its own induction process. Like AA, they effected major changes in their members' behavior, but clearly in a much more global way. Whereas AA focuses on alcohol abstinence, these movements addressed many more aspects of their members' lives.

These movements were effectively an experiment of nature begging to be understood. How did they exert their influence on large numbers of young adults? Some groups were of Eastern origin: the Divine Light Mission headed by a young guru from India, and the Unification Church led by Sun Myung Moon from Korea. Both groups engaged thousands of followers who lived communally and carried out the unique and strange practices they were expected to follow.

Beth, a friend of mine from college, had joined one such movement, The Divine Light Mission, and invited me to go to an ashram (a spiritual retreat) of theirs in Manhattan, actually not far from where I lived. Beth had been a thoughtful leader of student activities in college and a talented medical student. She first encountered the group while in a gap year waiting to transfer from an internal medicine residency to psychiatry.

While speaking with people at the ashram, I found the Mission's influence was quite remarkable. One woman, a heroin addict, had joined them and was now abstinent from drugs. Another, a chronic schizophrenic who had blinded herself with her own hands, was now sitting comfortably between two members and listening to a *satsang*, a ritual sermon. It seemed to me that the mutuality and support among members had somehow transformed these young people. I decided to see whether the nature of its influence could be subjected to research.

One important issue for studying these cultic groups, and equally important in the later study of the Twelve Step movement, is that a researcher needs to be sanctioned by someone whom members of the group can trust.

This can be based on an introduction from a long-standing member. That is to say, the group must see the researcher as someone who is safe to enter its envelope of mutuality, or cooperation will not be forthcoming. In this case, my friend from medical school was now working closely with the guru, and her introduction to the group's hierarchy created an option for me to carry out a study on the members.

My hypothesis was that distressed young people were somehow drawn in by the support of existing members who appeared caring and provided emotional support. Importantly, it appeared that the very experience of this support led to a relief in recruits' distress, generating involvement that yielded a compliance with the group's expectations. The relief from distress (I termed this a "relief effect")[1] and the resulting improved well-being would reinforce continuing participation and membership. By "reinforce," I mean to habituate (as in operant psychological conditioning). The expectations for membership were set by the leader, Guru Maharaj Ji, who had migrated to the States from India. These were instilled in a social setting where care and support could be felt intensely. Here is how the heroin addict who stopped using upon joining the Mission put it:

> Once I got to know them, I realized they loved me. They took me up, and it was as if they were holding me in their arms. I was like a baby whose mother guides its moves and cares for it. When I wanted to take heroin, or even to smoke [marijuana], I knew they were with me to help me stay away from it, even if I was alone. And their strength was there for me, even before I could hardly meditate at all. I could rely on their invisible hand, moved by Maharaj Ji's wisdom, to help me gain control.

Given the entrée we were accorded, a colleague, Peter Buckley, and I were able to attend a large conclave of the members in Orlando, Florida. After some lengthy negotiations, ultimately including clearance by the Maharaj Ji himself, we were able to administer a survey to attendees. It included psychometric scales for measuring the strength of their social ties toward other group members and measures of any change in mood they experienced upon joining. We found that the original hypothesis was validated.[2] That is to say, the more a recruit had come to feel tied in to established members, the more her or his mood had improved upon joining. The resulting idea was that in order to maintain relief from distress, they would need to stay affiliated, because a wavering in commitment could result in feelings of distress emerging. What this meant in psychological terms was that any questioning of commitment by a given member was an aversive stimulus, a discouraging pressure. Thus, there was a potentially negative emotional pressure to avoid feeling distanced from the group.

After these results were published, it occurred to me that an additional aspect of this movement was important in engaging these young people. It seemed reasonable that the degree to which they accepted the group's system of beliefs was reinforcing in the same manner as were the social ties to the group. The chance to assess this came about when I was later able to do research on the Unification Church (the "Moonies," as they were called). These followers of the Reverend Sun Myung Moon gave up their property to the sect and engaged in rituals that were shocking to members of the general public. They lived communally with shared clothing. They went out begging in the streets while being icily removed from talking with passersby. They participated in mass engagement and marriage ceremonies with hundreds of other members and were betrothed to whomever Reverend Moon seemed to arbitrarily match them. They were getting negative publicity in national media because they were said to be "brainwashed." The head of their U.S. national office in New York sanctioned a study of them on the assumption that any objective assessment of the members might allow the public to perceive them as less sinister.

A series of studies ensued, producing further findings on how the young adults joined the movement, and how their willingness to go along with its demands was stabilized. When young people encountered the group, as in the Moonies' workshops, the likelihood of a given person's joining was directly proportional to how distressed and alienated they had felt upon first arriving. That distress then apparently fueled their willingness to become involved with the members they were exposed to, and to accept their beliefs. Their relief was directly proportional to how much they accepted the group's beliefs and to how affiliated they felt toward other members.[3] Those who joined apparently became conditioned (habituated) and committed by their implicit need to maintain a positive mood.

The members I spent time with were indeed enthusiastic and positive about their involvement. The support and sense of purpose the Church gave them was striking. What all this meant, in effect, was that members' engagement and participation was fueled by the need to maintain a positive mood state, even though they might not be fully aware of this. Conditioned reflexes do not have to be consciously perceived.

Once they were engaged, members were put through disruptive and stressful experiences, but their affiliative feelings compensated for the distress these demands imposed on them.[4] They experienced a great deal of stress in numerous ways: giving up all their personal property, begging in the streets among hostile strangers, and giving up their choice of spouse to Reverend Moon. Their mutual support and beliefs, however, served to compensate for this by sustaining their spirits.

This body of research helped to develop a model that would shed light on the beneficial effects apparent in AA. The cultic groups could be considered "charismatic groups," or groups bound together by an overriding ideology that leads members to give up their place in life and adapt their "new" lives to the norms of the group and its charismatic leader. The followers of the Guru Maharaj Ji and Reverend Moon fell into this category.

On the other hand, a similar psychology can be evident in less intense settings. Among these are "spiritual recovery movements,"[5] which draw on the beliefs and affiliative feelings of members, but focus more narrowly on issues of recovery from illness. They do not usurp the freedom and autonomy of participants. These latter groups tend to arise when conventional medicine cannot resolve the health problems it is asked to address. Because of this, nonmedical approaches are sought out for recovery. The biggest such spiritual recovery movement in the United States in our time is AA, which emerged at a time when doctors had little, if anything, to offer despairing alcoholics in the way of recovery from their illness.

The most distressed alcoholics are the likeliest to join AA. It provides them a belief system couched in spirituality and a strong sense of mutual support, transforming those who are open to its message into followers who comply with the group's expectation to give up the idea of drinking. Their commitment to AA promotes and sustains a positive mood, even in the face of the stress of having to stay away from alcohol.

But AA does not control all aspects of the members' lives. They retreat to their own homes at night. They obviously keep their own property, dress as they choose, and marry whomever they wish.

There was another natural laboratory for dramatic transformations when I first began to study AA. It was not a charismatic group, in that it did not usurp the autonomy of its members, but it was a zealous movement that led "converts" to achieve a sense of personal renewal. Although this renewal could come about relatively suddenly, it was not a vision as in the case of the dramatic "white light" experienced by Bill W. It did, however, seem to represent a significant renewal. "Est" was an acronym for Erhard Seminars Training, led by Werner Erhard, a dynamic speaker with a background in sales. It offered well-educated adults the opportunity to attend two weekend-long workshops, with evening sessions on the intervening work days. Large numbers of participants, perhaps 200, would be lectured, even harangued about the need to change their lives in order to "transform their ability to experience living." Participants were confined in the meeting space and expected to stay in their seats. They were subjected to uncomfortably low temperatures, and prohibited from speaking with each other—all this while being exposed to established group leaders, or "trainers," as they were called.

Some participants responded with intense emotion, sometimes crying, or shouting their responses. At the end of the sequence, in the midst of a harangue, enrollees were asked, "Did you get it?" "Getting it" meant something particular for each enrollee. It related to achieving some transformation that they thought would put them in active control of their lives. Some said yes, others no. The "yes" participants left with what they felt was a new and vibrant outlook on life. This apparently showed that an immersive group experience could enlist a relatively sudden personalized and dramatic change. And the change in this case was not necessarily specific, but it still generated great zeal. Many alumni went to great effort to enlist their friends in "est." As we shall see with regard to spiritual awakening among AA members, dramatic transformations can come about if people engaged in a zealous group are led to expect their lives can be transformed.

Here is one salient point about all the intensely experienced changes we have discussed here. They took place in an era when psychiatry considered the line between unhappiness and euphoria to be part of a continuum, which, in its extreme, could verge on manic-depressive illness, where a person's feelings get out of control in a way that is considered pathologic. Some psychiatrists thought to pathologize the changes described in these cultic movements and to ascribe them to something akin to mental illness. A better explanation can be related to the writing of the psychologist William James, and specifically to his perspective on personal transformations described in his classic, *The Varieties of Religious Experience*:

> Medical materialism finishes up St. Paul by calling his vision on the road to Damascus a discharging lesion of the occipital cortex, he being an epileptic. It snuffs out St. Teresa as a hysteric, St. Francis of Assisi as a hereditary degenerate.[6]

In other words, dramatic transformations throughout history have to be considered in their own right when they relate to religious experience, and not be boxed into some conventional medical model.

Given this, let's step away from the more prevalent approach employed in psychiatry today, with its diagnostically grounded system, and consider how social settings can generate dramatic changes in people's thinking. When and how might this happen? Certain situations increase the likelihood that a person will be influenced by cues in her environment to adopt a new set of attitudes. As was described by the psychologist Harold Kelley, this is most likely to take place when the following three conditions are met, namely, when individuals:[7]

- feel little social support
- have prior information that is poor or ambiguous, and
- are confronting problems beyond their capabilities.

This is the kind of situation that the young members of new religious movements were in when they were being recruited. Those most likely to join were alienated, uncertain about their future, and uncertain what that future held for them. People came to est with dissatisfactions as well, hoping for answers. These young people and grownups could all undergo a transformation in their views—but so can the unhappiest of alcoholics who come to AA. They are primed to attribute their situations to a new perspective, and to acquire a new set of attitudes, and thereby find relief in their distress. Their relief is experienced as a new, presumably enlightened, positive state of mind of an awakened self. In the case of AA, a new member's uncertainties and distress are relieved by accepting the concept of abstinence and belief in a higher power guiding their lives.

Some people may find AA meetings useful and supportive, and that in itself can be helpful. For the people who become fully engaged, however, a greater transformation takes place. It can be as varied as there are members in the fellowship. This transformation depends on individual personalities, members' previous experiences, on the way their addictions played out for them, and on the circumstances of how they came into the fellowship.

THE AA MEETINGS

People are first introduced to the AA experience at the fellowship's regular meetings. How are these meetings set up? With some 50,000 of them held each week across the United States, they are, in practice, more available than are the churches of any major religious denomination. I point this out, not because AA should be likened to a religion, but because an addicted person need never feel that the fellowship's spirit and practice are far away. A member can find them almost anywhere they find themselves, on business, at home, or on vacation. In big cities, fellow members are available every day of the week at almost any hour. This alone offers a sense of security to a struggling alcoholic, with protection from vulnerability that can be very reassuring.

Most meetings are "closed." That is to say, they are available only to members, and not to outsiders who might compromise the anonymity of participants, and perhaps their ease in speaking up. There is a feeling of security in knowing that one can share experiences over which one might feel shame or guilt, but not to have to worry about enduring the judgments that members of the general public might feel about these experiences.

How protective is this virtual wall around closed meetings? I had one experience of inadvertently finding myself at a closed Narcotics Anonymous meeting. The NA World Services public relations director had suggested I go to the meeting as a way of getting a sense of how NA meetings compared to those of AA. (It turned out that the meetings were almost identical.) At the end of the meeting, a woman came over and would have welcomed me. When I told her I was not an addict, but a researching doctor who had been referred by some faceless "central office," she upbraided me for disrupting the security of the meeting. She might have been unduly inhospitable, but frankly, I felt mortified.

Not all reactions are like that one. While in Cuba, I was told by a physician who worked with addicts of an NA meeting conducted in Spanish. I went to the meeting in a rundown part of town, hoping to compare it to its American counterparts. (It too seemed little different from meetings Stateside.) When asked to identify myself, I explained that I treated addicted people, and was warmly received.

A minority of meetings are listed as "open," and non-alcoholic people—a spouse, a medical student, an interested community member—are welcome to attend. These meetings serve as a valuable resource for providing non-members with practical information about the fellowship, while at the same time alcoholic attendees know that outsiders might be present. Members are quite welcoming to the non-alcoholics who attend and they try to address whatever concern brought them there.

What is the atmosphere like in a typical AA meeting, a setting that can serve so effectively to engage its potential members? Even though many in the room find themselves among virtual strangers, they are not necessarily guarded about their troubles or failings, as they might be with non-members on the outside. A first-time attendee sees that those there, some like himself, and others not, have experienced and done things they regret, but nonetheless find acceptance among those present. In accord with AA culture, the tone is always accepting. Speakers are expected to be honest in what they are saying, and genuine expression is prized and expected. They only speak about their own experiences, and not about other members, and do not provide general information, religious dogma, or scientific theory.

People at the meeting will not intrude on a stranger but will, if he seems open to it, unobtrusively welcome him. If he is desirous of help to stay sober, they will give him their phone numbers, explaining that he can call them any time. In this way they adhere to what Bill W himself had found: The best way to introduce another alcoholic to sobriety is to tell him your own story, and not to exhort him about the path he should be following. This welcoming, nonintrusive atmosphere can provide relief to a confused or frightened person, even with no more complicated a message than encouragement to come back.

Here is how Ann, at wits' end, described such an experience. The daughter of a chronically alcoholic father, she had been afraid to drink at all through her college years, knowing what it might do to her. After college she began to socialize with people for whom drinking was the norm, decided to try it out, and very soon fell into two years of daily drinking, bouts of drunkenness that she could not later recall, and behaviors she deeply regretted.

One morning she awoke at the apartment of a man with whom she had gone to a movie the night before. As was often the case, she had no recollection of how she found herself there. Her date was gone and she was frightened. She called a friend and asked him if he thought she was alcoholic. He suggested she go to an AA meeting; maybe she would find out if she was while she was there. All she knew was that she was coming to hate what had befallen her. She looked up a nearby AA meeting, and describes here what she had said to herself at the time:

> "I think I'm going to an AA meeting tonight because they're the right people to tell me. And you know what, if they're not, then I'm going off the roof when I get home tonight." My biggest fear was, What if I'm not? What if I'm totally crazy? What if I walked in there and they said no, you're not an alcoholic, you're just nuts? It was my last hope, because I knew I could not go on living the way I was. I was so full of self-hatred and fear. I didn't know what this monster was that was living inside me, and I really thought I was insane. At the AA meeting that night, I had a little styrofoam cup and I remember tearing it to shreds, little itty bitty pieces and shaking, shaking, shaking, partly from withdrawal. I remember people saying, "Just come back; you're in the right place."

Ann did come back, and when she told me this, she had been in AA for some twenty years. She initially went to meetings almost daily, and now goes every week or so.

Here are some more examples of what makes for a feeling of safety at the meeting. There is no cross talk; people speak in turn, and no one interrupts or counters anything that was said. No one can convey that they are better or smarter than another person; one reason being that there is an understanding that no matter how long one has been sober, or no matter how secure one feels today, a slip or relapse could come tomorrow. Each speaker acknowledges that they cannot get away with drinking, and people who qualify begin with, "I'm Joe (Mary, Tom, or whoever), and I'm an alcoholic." In the fellowship that means that sobriety is the only answer for you.

AA meetings are different from group therapy. In group therapy, a therapist orchestrates the course of the therapy session, and does so without a fixed agenda. Group therapy participants never have to raise their hand to be called on, and can interrupt each other at times. They speak relatively briefly, and do not occupy a speaker's podium for ten, even twenty, minutes. Group therapy participants can be critical of one another, even express anger, and the anger may be interpreted by the group leader so that participants can learn to understand themselves better. They typically do not socialize outside the sessions and they have no sponsor to advise them how to proceed along any ritualized steps.

There can be exceptions to the safety that is usually the case in Twelve Step meetings. Young women are sometimes preyed on by older male members. This was publicly reported to have gotten to a very regrettable situation some years ago[8] in the Washington area, where the Midtown Group, with meetings held in various local churches, became cult-like, with teenage girls being pressured to sleep with older male members, and threatened with relapse if they dared to stop attending. By tradition, the AA General Service Office took no public stand on these meetings or any other meetings, given that groups are understood to be autonomous. Ultimately, the Midtown Group's meetings were dropped from the churches where they were being held. The phenomenon collapsed under the weight of mounting allegations and negative publicity.

VARIETIES OF ENGAGEMENT

We will now consider some examples of AA members, in order to illustrate how they became involved in the fellowship, each in his or her own way. Some joined under duress, some fortuitously. Some joined amidst the course of multiple relapses, and others never did fully join in.

Here is one example where a transformation was generated under pressure from an outside agency. For many college students, heavy drinking becomes an audition for later alcoholism. It can take place in a fraternity or among friends, but in either case a young adult can be enveloped in a culture where the norm is to get drunk regularly, at least on weekends. Murray is a fifty-eight-year-old oncologist who was already headed for problems with addiction while in college. He reported that,

> I started drinking heavily when I was the only pre-med in my fraternity. I studied hard and drank hard until I passed out doing shots, and I thought it was great. In medical school my drinking escalated and I started smoking a lot of pot and doing cocaine, but academically I was doing very well. During a [medical] fellowship after my residency, I didn't have any time on call and thought I could drink as much as I wanted, and the drinking escalated. When I came back as an attending, I started doing crack, and drank to come down.

Murray was driving his car one night while intoxicated, and he was stopped by the police. The incident was reported in his local newspaper, his medical license was put in jeopardy, and he was humiliated. He had no ally to turn to.

His situation resembled what the psychologist Harold Kelley had described: He felt little social support, had prior information that was poor or ambiguous, and was confronting problems beyond his capabilities. He was primed for accepting a new set of attitudes, but was still in the throes of denial. In order to save his license, he agreed to go to rehab by the State's Committee on Physician's Health (CPH). This is how he came to feel about the CPH at that time:

> They were dictating what I'd have to do. So I felt threatened by them. They had the power if they didn't like me to stop me before going back to work. It was a ridiculous thought, but when I came back to work I found them to be a support, someone in my corner when nobody else was in my corner. So they really cared. They want you to do well. Their interest is in a physician healing.

How did such a transition in attitude come about? Let's compare the AA-based rehab setting to which Murray was sent with the induction workshops where many of the Unification Church recruits were brought into the sect's fold. Although seemingly quite different, there are some important similarities:

The atmosphere was highly supportive in both settings. In the Unification Church, they called it "love bombing," and the AA meetings in rehab had a tone of caring and support. Long-term AA members worked as counselors, and because many were in Twelve Step recovery themselves, they were supportive and accepting.

- The nature of communication in each setting is set by group members already there, and these members express their belief system without ambivalence. In the Unification Church, induction workshop groups were set up so that most of the members explained their experiences in terms of their cultic world view. For example, inductees were encouraged to report their dreams, and the dreams were interpreted based on the Church's philosophy. In AA, a successful abstinent recovery produces relief from distress and results in a sense of well-being. In both settings, the established members put forth their creed with a sense of comforting certainty.
- The cost of relief is acceptance of the group's creed. In the Unification Church, it was the quasi-divine role of Reverend Moon. In the rehab, members can avow commitment to following the AA Steps, the first of which is: "We were powerless over alcohol—and our lives had become unmanageable."
- A recruit will achieve relief from stress and maintain a benign state of mind only if he complies with the expectations put forward by the group. In the Moonies, it was to carry out a number of rituals, like living communally and giving up traditional family ties. In AA, it is accepting a life of abstinence from alcohol and other drugs.

So as Murray could now say after years of AA membership, and after having worked all its Steps:

> You know, I believe in a power greater than myself. I don't think this is all about me. I believe there is a higher power, and I am here to do good, and that there is a purpose for me and that's why I'm still here. I don't think things happen arbitrarily. I think things happen for a reason, though we may not understand it. And this is the power that controls me.

What, in fact, is controlled by that higher power? In the Moonies, it dealt with all aspects of life, including having one's spouse selected by Reverend Moon. In AA it infringes most specifically on one issue, that of maintaining abstinence. When asked if he believed in a Higher Power before he went into recovery, Murray said:

The opposite. I totally didn't believe in any of that. What happened to you was the consequence of what you did. You were responsible. Good things happened because of my being smart. Bad things happened because I had bad luck. And there was nothing more powerful than myself.

Proselytizing was also an activity held in high regard by the Moonies, and in his own way, Murray carried out his Twelfth Step mission of "carrying the message" relative to his experience under the CPH program for addicted physicians.

You know, I'm extremely busy. I mean, if I were to tell you how busy I am, you'd probably be very surprised. I don't think there's anyone in [my community] who is busier than I am as an oncologist. But whenever I can, I give talks to doctors to let them know how much the CPH can do for them, and of course I serve as a sponsor in the [AA] program, too.

Murray's conversion was not to a traditional religious denomination, but rather to the AA system of beliefs. And his transformation was to the AA creed, rather than to a traditional doctrine.

I pray a lot. I often pray during the day. But I don't believe in religion. I was raised Catholic, but I don't practice my religion. I think that religion separates people a lot of the time. I don't go to church. I don't feel that my Higher Power is Catholic or Jewish or Muslim. It's just an omnipotent power. And I don't control what happens. It sort of helps me deal with things for reasons I may not understand.

Are all people vulnerable to—or capable of—such transformations? Likely they are, under the right circumstances.

Some Young People Join Age-Specific Groups

Murray, the doctor, went through adolescence drinking heavily, falling prey to excess only years later. That is the way many people manage to get by while their addictions are taking hold, perhaps with some bruises along the way. Nowadays, though, some young people do not make it that far, and may have to turn to AA in adolescence. In New York, there are now meetings for adolescents and young adults that the city's "Young People in AA" lists on its website. These include groups such as "Never had a Legal Drink," "Campus Cheer," and "Youth Enjoying Sobriety (YES)." One member of the YPAA leadership group told of his difficulties when he had been on the way to joining the fellowship while still in his teens.

Jack had been suspended from college after being charged with selling marijuana to support his own pot habit, and was now heading toward flunking out with finality.

> In high school, I drank to get wasted, but by college I was into weed. I was smoking literally from the moment I woke up till I went to bed, and was high pretty much round-the-clock. Then I was drinking and blacked out a few nights a week. I would try to stop pretty much every single day, and I would rarely last more than six hours. I think the longest that I ever didn't smoke since I started smoking was three days, and I was drinking during that time. But usually I would almost never last more than a few hours. I knew that my parents wouldn't pay for me to fail college again. And I would get high to escape the increasing tidal wave of problems. A lot of that feeling of dread, constant dread, was about where I was at school-wise.

Jack saw a substance abuse counselor at the college, but was not making progress. His introduction to AA came about unexpectedly, but the encounter apparently impelled him to begin to address his problem.

> The counselor invited me to participate in group therapy. One day after the group, one of the guys said to me, "Hey, do you want to go to a meeting? I haven't been in a really long time, and I would really feel more comfortable rolling with someone," and I was like, sure. My friend had assured me that I could be a fly on the wall, but when they asked if anyone was there for the first time, I said, "Hi, I'm Jack," and I think I said, "I'm an addict," but I didn't even think about stopping drinking. Weed was by far my priority.

Jack's despair had apparently primed him to grasp for the support he was offered. He was, as we said before, feeling unsupported, unsure of what to do, and confronting a problem that was beyond his capabilities to address.

The atmosphere in the group had drawn Jack in, even without his awareness of how this was coming about. It illustrated how a group of young people, acting as they might, resonated with someone of their own age.

> They were laughing and they were light-hearted. It seemed that they had moved beyond their problems. You probably don't have to go to AA unless you get to the point where you are unable to stop on your own, or by traditional

means. In a way, AA worked to a certain extent, because I was unable to stop any other way. My sober date was after my second meeting . . .

I don't necessarily think you have to be fully conscious about it before it can start to have an effect. Certainly I was not thinking about Higher Power and stuff after my very first meeting, but I think looking back on my experience in those early meetings, I kinda went to AA almost on autopilot. I just went to meetings almost robotically in the very beginning. I think part of it was because I had a really, really strong desire to stop.

Years passed, and Jack stayed faithful to AA, ultimately assuming elected offices in Young People in AA. He was focusing on using the Internet to disseminate information on the program. Although now established as a professional, he still maintained fidelity to helping people who were of the same age that he was when he joined.

Struggling to Connect

Murray the oncologist entered rehab and successfully connected with AA over weeks of rehab during which he was pressed to engage. Jack, on the other hand, responded to AA on his first encounters. For many AA members, however, perhaps most, there is a trail of failures at achieving abstinence before they finally succeed. They may go to meetings and, at first, see some value in them, but do not fully respond. (Some attendees, of course, never connect.) When AA members say, "Just come back," it is an acknowledgment that it can take time, and often repeated relapses, to fully enter the fold.

Karen had been a talented dancer in high school shows, and dropped out of school when she was given the opportunity to dance professionally. She was drawn into the world of alcohol and drugs while in the company of other entertainers, but found that she could not drink heavily without passing out.

The way I became an alcoholic was when I discovered cocaine—and when I used cocaine, I didn't get drunk. It was like the magic elixir that made it so that I could drink like everybody else. So for me the alcohol and cocaine went together.

She later married a man who would drink and use cocaine with her, but he would not be overtaken by their use. While first married, Karen could restrict her "partying" to weekends, but then she started using during the day while her children were in school. The drugs had captured her.

I did things I wouldn't imagine now. I would have slept with an elephant if I knew it would get me drugs. It was all about the party. I wanted to dance all night in the clubs. I was very, very skinny by the end, 5'9" and probably about 116 pounds. I was covered in bruises and I was very unhealthy.

My husband didn't like what this stuff did to me. He put his foot down one day and said "You know what? If you don't clean your act up, I'm gonna make you get outta this house." He was giving me orders to stop, and yet he was partying on in his own way.

And her husband wanted her to get high at parties, but just so far. Karen, though, realized she had a problem that had gotten out of hand when she began mismanaging her kids while high.

I just decided that if I didn't stop using all this stuff that my family and my children would be in danger. I went to an AA meeting. I was thirty, and everybody seemed like old farts to me. I saw that my life had become unmanageable, but I wasn't ready to give it all up yet.

It was six months after that meeting, while my kids were at school, that I checked myself into a rehab. I packed a bag and told my best friend across the street from me what I was doing. I said please, when the kids get off the bus, keep them and tell my husband he can't try to talk me out of it.

Her husband could not accept her giving up on their lifestyle, nor did he understand why she would dare to leave so abruptly.

And of course, my husband was right there that night and mad as he could be. He wanted me out. But there was no way I could control myself like he could. He could carry around cocaine in his pocket for two weeks and not touch it. I refused to leave and stayed there for twenty-eight days.

Like so many others who go to rehab, Karen had no professional follow-up, and no systematic way of channeling her confused state into positive action. She was destined to relapse shortly after leaving. There was continuing exposure to drugs and alcohol and continuing tension with her husband.

For the next 18 months after I got out of rehab, I really, really struggled. I thought I could still be cool and party with these guys and just not drink and drug. They could all drink and drug around me, but I'm not gonna use it. I just kept relapsing and relapsing. I was still going to AA and kept starting my day count over and over.

But she kept going to meetings now and then, knowing it was her lifeline.

> At one meeting, I said I would pick up because I would get jealous or angry at my husband for his behavior. Then someone at a meeting said to me, "Let me just get this straight. The most precious possession you have is your sobriety. You would take your most precious possession and throw it in the garbage because you are mad at your husband?" I listened to what she said and that was the day that I stopped drinking.

What had happened to Karen here? The pressure to use cocaine and to drink was creating an unmanageable tension for her, but her use was fueled by her anger at her husband. She was in a frightened and unstable state. The context of the AA meetings could offer support and a way out, but she needed just the right trigger to be transformed to turn toward a positive attitude and course of action.

Karen told me all this after seven years of abstinence. She was still married, even if the relationship was far from perfect. Her husband now used cocaine occasionally, and still drank a fair amount. The oldest of her children was now in college and out of the house. The other two were still at home. The household was not without tension, but Karen was committed to her sobriety.

While in Therapy for "Something Else"

Most psychiatrists do not specialize in addiction, and are inclined to refer alcoholic patients to someone who does. If alcoholism comes up in their sessions, it is often seemingly incidental to the problem the patients said they came to address. When it does come up, the patients will generally avoid talking about it or will minimize it. One reason for this is the denial that accompanies an addiction problem: "It's not really a problem." In addition, if they were to bring it up, they fear they might have to give up a habit that they find comforting, given that the doctor might see it as something that compromises their well-being.

Laurel, a newspaper reporter, was referred to me by a patient of mine who lived on the same floor in their apartment house. She did not present herself as an alcoholic: She was having trouble with a boyfriend who would neither accommodate her, nor go out of his way for her, nor regard her with respect. What she did not mention, was that she was always drunk when she spent time with him.

Her drinking came up after some time, and only peripherally, but it did seem to present a material problem. I told her I thought she might benefit from going to some AA meetings. She thought this unnecessary, so I suggested she go as a journalist, a reporter-observer: She could be researching it for possible material for her newspaper. Years later, this is how she described her journey to abstinence, and why for a long time she could not acknowledge the actual severity of her drinking problem.

> Like why it took me so long? The pain when my feelings would get hurt, and the loneliness just seemed unbearable without alcohol, and so I couldn't be honest about how much I was drinking, because I think I wanted to have the option to resort to it, if that makes any sense.

Laurel did, however, talk about how she felt uncomfortable just being herself if she was at a social event with people her own age. This was an issue for which she realized she needed help, and was not afraid to acknowledge it.

> One thing that we used to talk about was that I had to get all dressed up and do up my hair and everything if I was going to be in any social situation, and you would say, look, you can just be yourself, but I was afraid of just being myself.

Her drinking was entwined with an insecurity born out of a childhood where she was disparaged by her parents. In her mother's eyes, whenever a problem arose, like kids picking on her at school, it was she who was always wrong. She dreaded how her mother related to her, even now as an adult. Some time later in sobriety, she had learned to pray in AA. To explain her anxiety over her mother, she cited what one woman in her AA group had said: "When my mom starts talking, I start praying."

Laurel's unease at being herself was heightened by a series of relationships with men who found her attractive both for company and for sex, but she would become anxious when intimacy arose.

> I needed to be drunk when I had sex. Once I started putting together days of sobriety, I would go on a date and I didn't want to tell the person I was sober. So they would drink, and I would drink and go to bed with them. Or I would get upset about something and drink. That was another reason.
>
> . . . I mean you have to drink when you're with a twenty-three-year-old guy [She was thirty-four], because otherwise if you're not drinking, you have to think about why you are with a twenty-three-year-old and not focusing on your career and finding an appropriate partner. If you're not drinking, you have to do the real work of putting your life together.

Even though she went to AA meetings at my request, it was threatening to her to acknowledge the depth of her drinking problem, and the fact that she was regularly slipping. She could not bring herself to get a sponsor because that, too, would have meant facing up to what she feared to acknowledge.

> I didn't have a sponsor. I would talk to people. It just wouldn't be honest. I was honest with them when I was sober, but then I would relapse and I couldn't be honest about it.

There came a time, though, when she had to move on from hiding the issue to acknowledging it, but the vulnerability was still there. She told me,

> I didn't want to be honest with you. One time I saw you when I was high and you asked me if I had been drinking and I said no. But I had. When I really started to be honest with you about how bad the problem was, in conjunction with the AA meetings, is when I started to get better.
>
> At one point I had put together some time and I really liked a guy, and I went on a date with him and he never called me. I had put together four or five months of sobriety. And I drank for three days in a row. I remember I called you after the three days and I was completely honest about what had happened. And that's when things started to really improve, because I was honest with you, and I went to a women's AA meeting, and I really started to get serious about sobriety after that.

Laurel did work with a sponsor to achieve stable sobriety, although she never did complete all the Steps.

We spoke a year after our last session. She had maintained her sobriety, bolstered by a stable relationship she had achieved in a marriage where she felt content. Although she only went to meetings irregularly, she had a sponsee in another city whom she pressed over the phone to stay abstinent. She was now pregnant with her first child. Not all paths through AA are "by the Book."

Only Keeping In Touch

When AA counts its members, it gets a total of those in attendance on a particular day. Most who are at any given meeting are regular attendees who are long-term members, have had a sponsor, and have gone through the Twelve Steps with their sponsor (or sponsors). Many would report having had a spiritual awakening. One might ask who the others are. Among them are some who come a few times and do not return, perhaps benefiting from the introduction to the value of recovery, perhaps not. Some have been sent by health workers who have concluded they need to stop drinking. They will address their addiction problem by other means, or not at all.

Then there are people who operate on the periphery of the program, so to speak. Like Laurel, they may eventually engage to the point of achieving abstinence and adopt a positive and constructive adaptation. Some of these infrequent attendees have continuing problems with their own personal conflicts. They may stay sober, but do not move forward toward a positive adaptation. Would they have benefitted from a more fully engaged role in the program? Are they folks whom AA members call "dry drunks"—people who are abstinent but still carry all the other "failings of their disease"? Whatever the case, they have problems in making the best of a life while abstinent from alcohol or drugs. For someone who can explore with them what holds them back, these issues may come clear.

Mel had material psychological problems from an early age. Certainly much of this was characterized by a simmering anger developed in relation to his father, who was demanding and oppressive. Mel could recount the times, even as a young boy, that he would leave the family apartment fuming after bitter encounters with his father, who was verbally but not physically abusive.

Although he came from a seemingly stable, upper-middle-class background, and attended an Ivy League college, Mel got involved with cocaine dealers on campus, managing to avoid arrest when the non-student professional felons were indicted. His anger and his rebellious nature, along with an unwillingness to succumb to any authority, led him to refuse to testify against the major dealers, and resulted in his spending time in jail for obstruction of justice.

Mel went on to a successful career in rock music talent management through ties he had established with people with whom he had worked and taken drugs. This lasted several years until he collapsed under the burden of his own drinking and drug use. With outpatient treatment and attendance at AA meetings he achieved sobriety, but he was not able to re-establish himself with the degree of success he might have achieved. He was bitter and unhappy. He persisted in attending AA, but never became fully engaged, and participated in therapy only intermittently.

Mel understood his problems, and understood why he held back on fully undertaking the AA program, but he was constrained by his unwillingness to fully engage.

> That's part of my problem; I was never really a good AA participant. I approached it in the same way that I approach a lot of things, which is I overintellectualize

it. So I knew the AA talk very well, and I think I understand AA very well, but I never shared consistently. So whatever benefit you get from that, I never got. And I never made very many friends in AA. And I would qualify [speak at the podium], but not participate otherwise, and that felt good because that's like playing to my sense of uniqueness. It's like you get to be the star while you are qualifying, and it's OK if you are also a participant, but I was using it kind of like an ego stroke, instead as of a way of recording my progress.

In particular, complying with the limited authority of a sponsor was too much to accept for Mel, given the lifelong anger he felt toward his father, the aggressive authoritarian.

I've had people who were like sponsors, and I have pretty consistently over the entire time had one or two people in the program whom I was close to, but I never had a real sponsor.

Nonetheless, he did keep up ties with AA. His sobriety was important to him because he remembered how profoundly depressed he would feel when he was coming down from a cocaine run.

The first few years I went a lot. And then, I started to ease off. For another few years I went a couple times a week, and these days, I go once a week or less. But at least once a month.

I was picking up a lot of AA wisdom, but I don't know how much of it I was actually taking on board. And I also know that while you're in a meeting, you are not using. And there is something about meetings, that if you go to a meeting that day it seems as if you're much less likely to pick up. And I do not pick up.

Mel realized that he might have to address some of his personal problems if he became fully engaged with other members, stayed with a sponsor, and worked the Steps. But it was his very psychological limitations that kept him from doing this. Progression through the Steps can be salutary in resolving some of the problems of one's past, as can coming to be open with another person, one's sponsor. But Mel could not do this.

I stay in touch with AA. It can be uncomfortable because like I said, I still feel like I got most of the problems, and I undoubtedly have been to a much, much lesser degree than originally. But I still get into all kinds of conflict with people, I still have trouble holding a job, I still have trouble doing the things I know I ought to. Even though I don't feel like killing myself, I'm acting like a very depressed person.

Would Mel have overcome these limitations had he stuck with AA the way the program stipulates? Perhaps so, but the question is moot, as he could not bring himself to do it.

Certainly Some Addicted People Will Not Become Engaged

AA's meetings are open to any alcoholic who chooses to attend, but the Eleventh AA Tradition states that the fellowship "is based on attraction rather than promotion." This means that AA does not solicit or pursue potential members. So, many alcoholic people will come to a meeting or two, stick to themselves, and not come back. They may be greeted and welcomed, but they will not be pursued or solicited. They will be left alone unless they choose to participate.

Some find the meetings unappealing; others may like the atmosphere, but feel that AA is not pertinent to them. In order to understand the nature of this open door policy—open in both directions—it is useful to see how the policy plays out. One reason that many compromised addicted people may find the meetings unappealing is that speakers make clear that AA is a program of abstinence. When they do come for help at first, most alcoholic people do not want to give up their alcohol entirely, and harbor the wish or expectation that they will be able to drink less and with less ill-consequence. They may not have moved beyond believing that, "I can take it or leave it," or, "I'm only here to please my wife, to get her off my back."

Others may not feel very compromised by their drinking, and indeed, their lives may not be severely disrupted. For them the program, with its expectation of deep commitment, may, in the balance, be more than they feel is worth the effort.

Harry came to me out of mutual agreement with his wife. He had gotten very drunk at too many extended-family occasions and it was time to do something about it. He occasionally drank to excess at home in the evenings with his wife and children, but he did not drink more than appropriate at business social events. At the family social events, however, he would sometimes drink until he fell down bleary-eyed. This had happened enough times to precipitate his arrival at my office.

Harry's situation relative to abstinence was interesting in that it illustrated how influential a spouse can be in determining the outcome of a drinking problem. As I often do, when consulted on substance abuse issues, I saw Harry with family members who could put his problem in context. I also suggested that Harry go to a few AA meetings, which he did. He came back saying the experience was wonderful and very engaging; he was even awe-struck, but he said he did not see a need to go back.

And why was this? Two family members were indeed concerned about his drinking. His sister felt he had to stop. The occasional humiliation he caused the family was more than they should have to face. His wife, however, came from an Irish family of happy, heavy drinkers, and it became clear that she felt that no husband of hers could be respected by the clan if he were abstinent. Although never overtly opposed to it, she never came out clearly for him to stop drinking. AA's philosophy of abstinence did not fit into her family.

Although Harry's drinking was quite a problem, he was, therefore, never enthusiastic about not drinking. My view was that if he did not drink at all, he obviously would not have a problem with drunkenness, but his situation was not that severe, and the die was cast by his wife's attitude born out of her family's subculture. AA fell out of the picture, and Harry and I embarked on a course of helping him to limit his drinking to a level where there were no more episodes as bad as before.

Another patient, Calvin, did not feel he had much in common with the people at AA meetings, often a complaint of someone in denial. In his case, though, this was true in that he was able to cut back with help. He would come home on the commuter train, have a drink or two in the bar car, and then top that off with "a drink or two" over the course of the evening. He would end up asleep early in bed or on a couch in the living room. But Calvin was an earnest husband, a good provider, and actually responsive to his wife's concern over the gulf that had grown between them with his drinking. He agreed to uphold being abstinent for three months. We then set up a regimen whereby he would never drink at home, but only on outside social occasions, where he had been able to limit his drinking. This plan seemed to work for him, at least for a time.

In both of these cases, these men's drinking was manageable with a measured approach to how much each might consume, namely through controlled social drinking—or so it seemed while we continued to meet. These two men may not have reached a point in the evolution of their drinking where it could not be controlled. Perhaps neither had the biology nor the psychology of someone whose alcohol problem would inevitably lead them to a downhill course that could only be modified by cutting alcohol out entirely. I have no follow-up on either of them.

What emerges from all these examples is that there is a diverse set of possible encounters with AA. This is not without considerable impact for a treating professional or family member who may stand by waiting for a change in behavior. For someone treating an addicted person, it means that no single formula or approach can apply across the board in referring a patient to the program. Ideally, a doctor would be able to keep in touch with a given patient over time to optimize what AA could do for that individual. For an addicted person or her family member, it means that one needs to understand how a person may respond to the option of attending AA, while remaining fully aware that a single referral may only be the beginning of a longer course of encounters with the program. In all cases, patience, understanding, and persistence on the part of all parties involved are called for if one is to become engaged in AA to effectively promote recovery. But this is true for any treatment of addiction.

CHAPTER 5

The Steps

When Bill W and Dr. Bob met in Akron, Ohio in 1935, the concept of a worldwide fellowship was hardly on their minds; they were just struggling to stay sober. But soon they began to recruit fellow alcoholics to stop drinking. Bob did this in Akron where he lived, and Bill in New York. Over the next few years it became apparent that there was a need to define a path for new recruits to follow, and the idea of reporting the experience of early members in book form seemed to be a good way to do this. The book was titled *Alcoholics Anonymous*, and this would later become the name of their emerging fellowship; members of AA would refer to as the Big Book.

The Oxford Group, a Christian revivalist movement, the nexus out of which the cofounders initially came, provided members with steps for a progression they could pursue. When Bill started writing the book, he drew up six steps that were based on what he had learned at Oxford Group meetings; after correspondence and phone calls with Dr. Bob, these were extended to twelve steps. The idea was to lead members toward a spiritual orientation as they worked their way toward recovery. We will review all the Steps here in some depth, as they make clear how AA members can progress within the fellowship, among those who do.

The nature of the Steps is transmitted through reading the Big Book and is reviewed at AA meetings; new recruits also are guided through them by an established member, a sponsor. This relationship is implied in the Fifth Step: "Admitted to God, to ourselves, and *to another human being* the exact nature of our wrongs." I have italicized the phrase to make its importance clear, as the concept of working the Steps with the guidance of an AA sponsor emerged from this, and over the decades new members have sought out sponsors with whom they felt comfortable to engage in this ritual.

These Steps embody the basic creed of the fellowship, namely, that members must turn to a Higher Power to address their alcoholism because they cannot overcome it on their own. It serves as the basis for fulfilling the ensuing Steps, which are designed to secure sobriety and to move toward a spiritual awakening. These first three Steps require a leap of faith that can be much harder to take than simply carrying out a specific set of tasks. Few, if any, people are prepared to do this upon first encountering AA, and frankly, few fully understand at first what they are getting into. Many will go to AA, and benefit from its support, but not become fully engaged at this level.

New members do not start working the Steps until they have substantial experience in attending the fellowship's meetings and have acquired an identification with other members. At that point, they may be encouraged by people they have met in the program, perhaps even a meeting chair or, for some, their therapist, to select an established member with whom they feel comfortable to serve as their sponsor. Most sponsors, who themselves have worked the Steps, will have their sponsee undertake this progression, usually the same way that they themselves had carried it out with their own sponsor. It is a ritual handed down from each generation of members to the next.

The labor of working these steps can vary greatly among various sponsors and sponsees, but let's look at how this played out for one woman as she undertook the First Step. As a college student, Betty had been studying in London, and began to drink quite heavily there. After she graduated, she came back to the States, where she began working in public relations, and where she progressed to heavy substance use.

> I was going out partying, doing coke in the morning instead of drinking coffee, and held my job together by a thread, but basically there were times that I would go in to work where I hadn't even gone home the night before, because I was out drinking until 6 or 7 in the morning. And I actually let go of my job and decided that it was just fate that I was supposed to figure out what I wanted to do next. I thought I wanted to work in music and work with bands, but really I was just partying. It was eight years of my drinking and drugging.

The First Step reads, "We admitted we were powerless over alcohol—that our lives had become unmanageable." This Step was designed to cut through the denial regularly experienced by the alcoholic, who can forget just what her addiction was actually like. Betty's sponsor required her to spell out the particulars of her addiction, effectively making something of a confession, and to face these—not only alone—but with her as well, being, in effect, "another human being," as described in Step Five.

> The specific work that I had to do was writing out my entire drinking and drugging story. For me, that was really helpful because it brought to light a lot of the things that I did, that might not have seemed so bad at the time. But when you really look at it, or think about it, what sane person would do that?

Acknowledging unmanageability might seem to put Betty, the alcoholic, in a helpless position, with no capacity to work toward a course of abstinence. It is here that the Second Step embodies an acceptance that she, along with other AA members, "Came to believe that a Power greater than ourselves can restore us to sanity" (Step Two). This clearly requires new members to negate the assumption that they can be wise enough to manage their sobriety with the usual resources they summon up to run their lives. After all, they have caused themselves and others great damage by relying only upon their own will. So here is how Betty undertook this Second Step for herself:

> What I realized from that Step is that in the years I had of partying, I always felt that there was something that was going to make things OK. Like there was something taking care of me whatever it was, like the universe's energy. And doing the Second Step made me be able to put a finger on it, or at least to name it, and I realized it was my God.

Here are some other examples of the varying ways these Steps can play out. Dan, an executive in a utility company, was undertaking the First Step. For him, drinking itself did not encompass the full impact of his illness. His family was in disarray; he had lost many friends; and he could barely hold on to his job.

> All I knew was that I was told that I had to stop drinking, but my sponsor started pointing things out to me and he also related some things about his own experience that I started to understand. Somewhere along the way this light bulb clicked on and I got it. I realized that my drinking was just a part of the unmanageability of my life before I made it into the rooms of AA.

The Second Step embodies coming to believe in a "Power greater than ourselves." Many people are turned off by this: "It's a religion," "It's a cult." Here are two ways that a person might accommodate to the Higher Power concept. The first illustrates how a woman, uncomfortable with the idea of "God," responded to this Step.

> I remember I had a real hard time when I came into the rooms hearing the word God. And then I started using Higher Power and hearing Higher Power. But I remember somebody saying to me, and I kind of clung to this for a while in the beginning, "It doesn't matter who your Higher Power is, as long as it isn't you. If it has to be the group, it can be the group of AA, or anything you can believe in, whatever it is that keeps you coming."

The latitude in that advice gave her entrée into the program without raising her hackles.

On the other hand, most Americans do have an affinity for the concept of God, usually from their religious backgrounds, and this can serve as a bridge to accepting the Second Step. Dan, the executive, still retained a commitment to his religious background and often attended church. Sometimes he would go to the empty church and just reflect. His relationship to the church made taking this Step easier for him.

> I referred to the God of my understanding as the God of my youth. I attended Mass regularly, thought seriously about joining a religious community, and admired religious people. Now, I accept that God, but I exclude any kind of notion that He is going to punish me if I don't go to church.

The Third Step carries the role of one's Higher Power further, and requires its own leap of faith: We "made a conscious decision to turn our will and our lives over to God as we understood him." Bill W pointed out, "No matter how much one wishes to try, exactly how can we do this?"[1] Indeed, when Bill spelled out the intent of the Third Step in *Alcoholics Anonymous*, he expressed the full intensity of the belief he felt through a prayer: "God, I offer myself to thee—to build with me and do with me as Thou wilt . . . May I do Thy will always!"[2] Bill does, however, acknowledge that, "The wording was, of course, quite optional so long as we expressed the idea, voicing it without reservation."

There are many workbooks that detail questions for a member to fill out while working each of the Steps. Here are some questions that may be asked for this Step: "What are your biggest fears about giving up control over your life to God?" "How do you think that you should live your life after giving up this control?" "What does 'the care of God' mean to you?"

Betty, the young woman who had hopes of working with bands, had to write everything in a notebook (no computer to depersonalize it) and read it over to the phone to her sponsor. After the Second Step, though, the Third did not seem like a great leap for her. She decided to let God take over, and found this comforting.

> Every single time that I would get myself into a corner or hit a wall, I had to let go to Him and see what would happen. Everything would sort of unfold for the better. And I would somehow miraculously just get out of whatever terrible situation I was in.

On the other hand, Dan was able to reach back to a modified version of his religious background.

> I had slowly developed a personal relationship with the God of my youth. In the early stages when I did Step Three, it was perfectly acceptable to me to believe in my heart and soul that turning my will and life over to God meant paying attention to AA's suggestions as though they were coming directly from God.

Some Perspective on These Steps

Working the Steps consolidates the induction of a new member into the fellowship. It entails acquiring a new personal philosophy and developing patterns of behavior that perpetuate abstinence. Bill W's "white light" experience transformed him suddenly. The psychologist William Miller described this as yielding a "quantum change," by which one's value system is turned around, not just modified.[3] But most AA members achieve a change in their values in a measured way, and this involves working the Steps over time, which in the end may lead to their "spiritual awakening." The process, however, is counterintuitive, which is to say that following these Steps entails going against the grain of one's natural inclinations, namely, that one is in control of one's life, and it is this very paradox that may take months to overcome. Consider the first two Steps that we have just discussed. Bill W elaborated on them in his book, *Twelve Steps and Twelve Traditions,* and spelled out what they were like in some detail. Here are some of his comments on them:

Step One. We admitted that we are powerless over alcohol—that our lives had become unmanageable. In describing this, he wrote, "Every natural instinct cries out against the idea of personal powerlessness."[4] As you can see, Bill himself was wise enough to realize what a leap of faith this entailed.

And then Step Two: "Came to believe that a power greater than ourselves can restore us to sanity." Bill follows this with, "Some of us *won't* believe in God, others can't, and still others who do believe that God exists have no faith whatever that He will perform this miracle."[5] Another leap of faith is required. And we could follow paradoxes like these all the way through the ensuing Steps.

What examples can we draw on to understand how attitudes can be radically altered? One way was described in the process of "brainwashing," originally studied by Robert Lifton to explain how some American soldiers who were prisoners of war in North Korea came to turn against their own country and voluntarily testify against it.[6] Some did this even to the point of fabricating war crimes that would serve as evidence against their fellow countrymen.

Some aspects of the brainwashing process that Lifton spelled out could be considered in relation to AA. One is the "cult of confession," namely an obsession with confessing, and thus relieving the growing guilt that was repeatedly instilled by one's captors. As we will come to see, confession of ills is part of the program of the Twelve Steps. In part of the Fifth Step, members must acknowledge "the nature of our wrongs."

Secondly, under brainwashing the group's precepts are considered to be sacred truths, which implies that they cannot be questioned because they have an absolute validity. In AA, of course, the whole program is premised on relinquishing one's judgment to a "Higher Power," a God-like figure who out of necessity validates what AA expects of a member. Once a deity, as it were, is embodied in the fellowship, its precepts cannot be questioned.

There is, however, a crucial difference between the brainwashing process that Lifton described and induction into AA. As the fellowship's Eleventh Tradition spells out, the fellowship's appeal must be one of "attraction rather than promotion." This makes clear that one can choose to look to a Higher Power for guidance—but in relation to AA itself, the individual's independence and decision to join lies in her own hands. Any AA attendees are free at all times to come or go, although they are always welcome.

On the other hand, stages of noncoercive religious conversion have been described this way: The psychologists Lewis Rambo and Steven Bauman[7] point out that after initially interacting with members of the group, inductees reach a stage when they commit to the group. This can take place in the context of a testimony or a ritualistic ceremony. Clearly such ceremonies are part of many religions, and in the case of Alcoholics Anonymous, there are rituals as well: regular meeting attendance, sponsorship, qualifying (speaking before the group), receiving tokens on the anniversaries of one's sobriety, even what one says when one first speaks to the assembled group ("I'm Joe, and I'm an alcoholic.").

Clearly, many people are put off by the concept of powerlessness over alcohol and then needing to turn to God. This includes many mental health professionals whose goal is to use psychotherapy to help patients recognize their drinking triggers and then learn to avoid acting on them, an approach that works for many alcoholics who are not so compromised that they are unable to do this reliably. For the most severely disabled though— those who are most likely to turn to AA—the fellowship provides a more intensive approach that may be necessary to their recovery. Because their drinking may indeed be unmanageable, a regimen of recognizing triggers may not suffice for them to avoid relapse. Engaging the support and ideology of the fellowship may be necessary. Additionally, their lives may be in such disarray that reclamation on a larger scale, such as working through all the AA Steps, may give them the chance at renewal that they sorely need. Even according to the psychiatric diagnostic criteria, the volume of alcohol or drugs consumed is not a criterion for diagnosis, but rather the disabling aspects of the disease. Damage to the psychological, interpersonal, and physical aspects of life is necessary for diagnosis.

And where can these three Steps leave someone after years of sobriety? Here is Murray, the oncologist who had been stopped by the police while driving high on cocaine. He had only joined AA after going to rehab under threat of losing his medical license:

> I couldn't tell you how it works. It just works. You couldn't tell me that I would never use alcohol or a drug for this last thirteen years. I would bet anything against it. I believe in a Higher Power. I pray a lot, too. I pray often during the day. I say the Serenity Prayer frequently. I take things and put them in my Higher Power's hands. It's a relief actually.

Steps Four through Seven: Character Defects

One member said,

> My sponsor pointed out to me that every time I talked about things that I did wrong, I would add 'because of.' I would explain why I did these things. And that was my continuing problem that I had with pride. I couldn't just say I did something wrong, I had to explain and rationalize.

The Oxford Group's principles included, "We got honest with another person, in confidence."[8] For them this meant sharing "sins and present temptations," because these were understood to stand between a member and

God. In making use of what he had learned from that revivalist group, Bill W formulated Steps that would ensure relief of one's failings after one made the decision to open oneself up to the "care of God." Steps Four and Five spelled this out as follows:

Step Four reads: "Made a searching and fearless moral inventory of ourselves." And Step Five reads: "Admitted to God, to ourselves, and to another human being the exact nature of our wrongs."

These Steps require a level of self-examination that is certainly not typical of most addicted people, who usually do not dwell on their own failings. If they were to open up to such issues, they might compromise the mental barriers they need to maintain to avoid responsibility for the many problems their addiction had brought about.

These two Steps entail looking at oneself with a new openness. They also underline the addicted person's acknowledgement of his guilt before another person, namely, before his sponsor. This implies a measure of subservience toward the sponsor that is compatible with a willingness to accept the expectation of abstinence and renewal represented. In order to carry out these two Steps, the sponsee lists those persons to whom she bears resentment. She then reflects on this and considers what "defect of character" of her own contributed to the problem. This expectation is often hard to face. To facilitate it, workbook questions can run something like this: Are there things you wish you could do over with your friends, family, and co-workers? Have you ever felt self-righteous? Explain when, and the circumstances. Was this fully justified? When reflecting on your detractor's failings, do you have any of these traits yourself?

Betty, whom we saw writing in her Step workbook, described her struggle with this task, and gave me this example:

> A person that I was resentful toward was my business partner, like number one on the list. There are certain things that I am very resentful over that she does. I feel like she is manipulative, and kind of embellishes the truth, and is insensitive in certain ways.

But then she had to look at herself as an actor in this situation:

> And what was my role in this relationship? My part in it was allowing her to control and to manipulate. There was a lot of hypocrisy, because I was doing a lot of the things that I was resentful of her for doing. One of the big things that I was resentful about was her using people or like socially climbing, but I was guilty of that as well.

The resentments that are exposed as one carries out this inventory can go back many years. Depressed people often ruminate about past wrongs, but even the nondepressed can summon up memories of past actions they regret, as could Dan, the retired executive, in the course of this Step:

> I remember a girl had broken up with me in high school, and I was quite angry about it. I had made some comments to this guy that I was friends with about the way she wasn't a good kisser. And he went back and told her, and she ended any relationship we had. I was really pissed off at him. But it shows me that I was talking negatively behind someone's back in order to be accepted by a friend.

Spelling out one's character defects to another person, one with whom a sponsee has social interaction, can be awkward. It still is essential to the process of carrying out these Steps, however, forcing a sponsee to confront the reality of his acknowledged failings. Dan described how this played out for him. Initially, he felt it would be easier to do this in a religious setting.

> I planned on doing my Fifth Step with a priest or a monk rather than my sponsor because I said to myself, my sponsor's a young guy; he's never been married and I had a twenty-year marriage. But I realized that this was my problem, because he was very trustworthy, and he was very supportive. So, we went to a very quiet spot on the grounds of this monastery, away from any possible distraction, and he gave me his undivided attention. My first thought was that maybe I don't have to read everything I wrote, which was just my desire not to reveal certain embarrassing moments, the infidelities particularly. But he made it very conversational. He opened up about himself more than he ever had. We were pretty honest.

These steps do open up an exchange between sponsor and sponsee about the meaning of the honesty that is expected of AA members.

The experience of Jared, a twenty-two-year-old who had been multiply addicted to pain killers and cocaine, sheds light on why it can be hard for a person to undertake these Steps. It also makes for an interesting example of how working the Steps can open up psychological issues that come up in therapy.

Jared had left rehab eleven months before, had attended AA reliably, and had worked the first three Steps with his sponsor with earnest resolve. He was reluctant, though, to take on Step Four because he realized that he was still holding on to the need to rationalize the consequences of his "defects of character" rather than face them. He acknowledged this in admitting that his abstinence, although stabilized, was not yet premised on being prepared to continue beyond Step Three. For one thing, Jared was still relying on family resources rather than assuming responsibility for himself.

> Like I came into the rooms and created a new life for myself, with the clothes and the money, the cool car and the job with my dad, and all that. I had jumped in head first and wanted to change everything overnight.

If he were to start his Fourth Step, he would have to list the resentments he bore toward people and then write down what role he had played in these. His old girlfriend Denise would have topped the list.

> I've been putting off my Fourth Step for so long. And I definitely think it has a lot to do with the fact that I'm afraid of looking at a lot of the things that I'd probably end up talking about. I would get angry at Denise because I wanted to go get high and she didn't know about it and she just wanted me to be there for her and hang with her. She had no idea because I had kept it hidden that I was a drug addict. I was in the wrong because the only reason that she would constantly nag me was that I was always trying to run away but I was really using coke, although I told her it was because of my 'friends.' In her head she obviously had some type of feeling like I didn't want to be with her. I didn't tell her the truth, probably a lack of patience and empathy. But I am not ready for that whole list. It's too much to take on.

Jared's need to deal further with his conscience was apparent in how he handled responsibility for his actions. One day, he inadvertently gave an example of this in a therapy session:

> I got a ticket today. I was in the fast lane and I had to get over three lanes to get off at my exit. There was a big truck to my right so I sped up and cut across the lanes. And there ended up being a cop right there. So he pulled me over and I got a ticket for reckless and aggressive driving.

He continued, explaining how he handled this upon coming home and speaking with his mother.

> I said to her, I got a ticket, it was for reckless driving and you know, I don't know what the points are. I think she said, Oh boy, and you're going to have to fight it. That was what she said. Something like that, and I agreed.

When I pointed out to him that he was more concerned with avoiding responsibility than with a need for contrition (or respect for the law), he acknowledged why the Fourth Step was intimidating. He would have to face that character defect.

> My mom doesn't want to see that I did something wrong just as much as I don't want to see it. And then I said to myself that I've got to get a radar detector because then I will be able to detect when these guys are around so I don't drive fast. Well I definitely see from breaking this down that I still obviously have an issue with taking responsibility for things when I do something wrong. I definitely didn't go home and think that you really need to slow down your driving and be careful because you could hurt somebody.

Jared was on the way to facing up to his character defects, but not quite there yet. The whole exchange also revealed his tendency to adopt a mode of manipulation as he was growing up in his family.

Having conducted an internal search, and having laid out his failings and bared himself to a sponsor, a sponsee is now dealing with vulnerability and guilt. He is ready to turn to his Higher Power, yield to Him, and achieve some comfort in His presumed forgiveness, as follows:

Step Six reads: "We were entirely ready to have God remove all these defects of character. Step Seven reads: "Humbly asked Him to remove our shortcomings."

This experience can be comforting because it can relieve a longstanding burden. Dan, the executive, described what happened with his anger in high school.

> I was going to relive the resentment I had toward this kid in order to get rid of it. If I give it to God, God is going to take care of it. By that, I mean I'm going to feel good about myself, because I'm giving it away to someone greater than myself to take care of.

Another member said,

> I know I felt good doing it and I felt like a part of the human race more. Turning that stuff over and getting rid of that yucky stuff, I was proud of myself.

This expiation can, therefore, be experienced in a positive way, one which some members continue pursuing over the course of later years in order to assure that they will maintain the honesty that they believe the program expects of them:

> I always kept a journal, even throughout my drinking and drugging days, so writing about my life hasn't been that hard. I always believe in writing and I believe

the writing is very healing. And I still do it. I'm not like some people in AA who say, "Oh I couldn't stand to write my fourth step." I was glad to be writing.

A Perspective

The ritual of examining one's own failings and seeking relief from God (as we understood Him) clearly suggests a comparison to the Catholic practice of confession, which dates back to antiquity. Some early Christians were subjected to persecution and torture by Roman emperors to the point of denying their faith in Christ. Those who came back to the church were called confessors, and asked for forgiveness for having denied their faith.

A classic example of confession is found in the autobiography of St. Augustine, written in the fourth century. Augustine was a Roman who was educated in pagan beliefs and who later converted to Christianity. In maturity, as he looked back over his life, he recalled acts that he attributed to his sinful nature, and over the course of thirteen books, *The Confessions*,[9] he recounted his transition to Christian redemption.

Although Protestants do not practice confession along these lines, confession was promoted by members of the Oxford Group. Founded by a Protestant missionary in 1921, the Oxford Group was accepted widely, even by the British Anglican church. The group's practice included confessions, which, interestingly, could be shared among group members, or alone with just one other member of the movement. And, indeed, Bill W modeled some of the Steps on the practices of the Oxford Group.

We can consider components that are typically part of the process of confession,[10] and these can be laid out in generic terms in relation to the Steps. First, there needs to be an accusation, which can be overtly stated or implied. In AA, a new member frames this accusation himself. The accusation also has to be backed by some measure of authority, and in the case of the Steps, that authority is invested in the process as explained in the Big Book, and under the eyes of a sponsor. There also needs to be evidence behind the accusation, and here again, the AA initiate himself is expected to provide that evidence, which can be written out in a notebook or in a Step-oriented workbook.

The accusation also has to be understood as coming from an authority with some power, one presumed to have some measure of a friendly role in relation to the accused. This is necessary for the accusation to have credibility, and here one's Higher Power and the fellowship itself serve this purpose. The confessor also must have some measure of guilt, and the Steps are premised on an assumption that the sponsees must write out their "defects of character," which they themselves acknowledge to have credibility. And finally the confession should yield some measure of freedom from the guilt the confessor bears, and indeed within the AA ritual, this liberation from guilt is afforded by one's Higher Power.

The psychoanalyst Carl Jung, with whom Bill W corresponded, had made some observations about the role of Catholic confession. He pointed out that this ritual breaks through the moral isolation that an individual may experience. In this manner, it can relieve the guilt a person suffers from that is associated with secrets, which may be apparent or even unconsciously borne.[11] By implication, these are circumstances from the past of which the confessor may not even be aware unless they are dredged up through a process like psychoanalysis. In AA, this takes place in Steps Four and Five.

Jung also made the interesting observation that when Protestants relinquished the ritual of confession in their religious practice, they left open a need that might be fulfilled in his lifetime by psychoanalysis. Jung was familiar with the Oxford movement, and pointed out that its emergence also addressed this psychological need, which had been left unfulfilled in the Protestant culture. In this respect, confession and forgiveness are located where psychology and religion intersect, that is, in the way they bear on how we deal with guilt.[12] This is evident in the rituals associated with Steps Four through Seven. An AA member who earnestly feels they have fulfilled these Steps can feel relief, even rejuvenation.

A different perspective on confession has been described by anthropologists[13, 14] who cited examples where confession serves to allow individuals to place themselves firmly within the social context of their cultural group, with examples of this drawn from East African rituals. Such examples may seem remote from New York and Akron where AA was formulated, but they illustrate the universality of confession rituals. In one, confession precedes the primitive ceremony of female circumcision. It involves confessing one's "social debts," which are essentially the refusal of other tribe members' requests. By means of these confessions, a girl cleanses herself and is then forgiven and inducted into the adult community with the ritual circumcision.[15] Another East African example involves a ritual ceremony where all participants shout out their confessions in unison. This is understood to validate their born-again Christian identity, relieves them of their "heathen" background, and brings them into the Christian community.[16]

Interestingly, both of these perspectives on confession, relief of guilt and incorporation into the larger community, can be seen to apply to the AA ritual of acknowledging one's own character defects. As we have seen, this allows sponsees to put their wrongs behind them and at the same time become further engaged in AA membership.

Although the Oxford Group provided a template after which Bill W and Dr. Bob could develop their fellowship's Steps, they realized that their own members had a unique quality that not all Oxford members had: Most had materially harmed people close to them over the course of their lives in addiction. Acknowledging one's defects of character could not in itself wipe the slate clean so that members could move forward with a feeling of forgiveness. They had to somehow face those whom they had wronged, and acknowledge what harm they had done. So here were two more Steps:

Step Eight: "Made a list of all persons we had harmed, and became willing to make amends to them all."

Step Nine: "Made direct amends to such people wherever possible, except when to do so would injure them or others."

In practice, this pretty much means apologizing, even trying somehow to make up for the harm done. If as a child you ever had your mom make you apologize for something she thought to be wrong, you can see this is not easy to do. Or perhaps you have had to get your own child to make such an apology to a teacher, a friend, or someone's parent. AA members now have to do this for a whole series of people whom they have wronged. This is a difficult, but potentially soul cleansing, experience.

Betty was working in public relations, but she had yet to go beyond Step Four and was anxious about taking on Step Eight. She pretty much realized what it would entail. Her experience also illustrated how a sponsor could help an uneasy sponsee with this:

> The idea that I had to face all these people that I had done wrong to, it terrified me, and I did not want to do it. There's a boyfriend I dated for three years and I cheated on him the whole time. And now I have to admit it to him, I just don't know what's going to happen. That's something that my sponsor would have to go through with me after I make those lists, and then we'll talk it through. My boyfriend was an addict. I didn't want anything to cause him using or relapsing. So that's what I was thinking, but my sponsor helped me to see it this way: Don't think about future steps until you get to them.

Betty's sponsor also reminded her that one does not make amends in a way that might do harm. Betty said this allayed her concern about these two Steps.

On the other hand, some AA members recall the process of making amends in a positive light, and with a sense of relief. Josh was a congenial and engaging person, and had been successful as a freelance art director until large amounts of cocaine tempered by alcohol and alpra-zolam (Xanax) had left him isolated from friends, and had compromised his professional contacts. He recalled being miserable and suffering from panic attacks as his addiction continued. A friend recommended that he go to AA, and from the outset Josh saw AA as a means of finding relief. AA meeting attendance, therapy, and medications were in the end respon-sible for his life turning around. By the time he was working the Steps, he reported his making amends was a positive experience.

> I've heard stories of people running into problems with people, but almost all of my amends, and I probably did thirty of them, were done in person. Some people told me that I hurt them or I worried them pretty significantly, and that kind of makes me feel a little bit ashamed, but I don't think I had one bad amends where someone was really angry at me.

Perhaps he had not, in fact, caused material compromise to people other than himself, or maybe he was somewhat superficial in his approach. He even recalled the experience with his mother quite fondly:

> The big one I made was with my mom. She was so proud of me being sober, and I had drawn up the list of things that I recalled that caused her great worry. It could be anything from not showing up at the train station where they were going to pick me up in my home town because I was still doing drugs. Just being honest with her about the things I had done and how they might have caused her pain was a relief. It was a really amazing experience. She was really incredible. She was great. She said, "Listen, we all make mistakes, and part of life is moving forward. And let's move forward from here."

Clearly, some people do feel great remorse for their actions while addicted, particularly in relation to their children, whose dependence on them for a stable home life may have been severely disrupted. Karen described how she had "partied" with coke and alcohol, often while her husband was at work. She had finally relented and decided herself to go to rehab, much to her husband's consternation. She described how she tried to make up for her behavior with her amends to her young children.

> I took each of them out and told them I was an alcoholic and that I can never drink again, and I had done some things when I left them with a babysitter I shouldn't have. I told them that I should have been home more during the weekends; it was very important to me that the kids go to their grandpar-ents on the weekends, because I wanted to party. They loved going to their

grandparents, so it was a perfect thing, but I'm sure after a while, the kids began to wonder why we're never home with Mom on the weekends.

Although Karen found this to be a relief of sorts, rather than too painful, some particular events a recovering person may remember can leave them feeling most remorseful. She recalled this:

> I felt very guilty about my youngest daughter because she mostly stayed with me in the house. I'll never forget one year, on her fifth birthday, I had had too much to drink and I was excited about her. I smacked her on her butt a couple of times. It was only playful, but I hit her too hard and she started to cry. I hurt her. I made amends to her, but she didn't even remember it.

Not everyone making amends is so easily forgiven: Anna had become addicted to heroin at an early age, and had gone onto methadone maintenance as a replacement for heroin. Her drinking, however, did not abate, and she ended up in a detox unit. Eventually, through persistence in AA, she gave up her drinking and slowly and painfully tapered herself off the methadone. Her son, though, did not grow up without scars from the experience of having a mother who bore him while she was still addicted.

> My son was born on methadone. I was twenty-two when I was pregnant. I didn't even know I was pregnant. I got sober when he was seven, so I kinda did a lot of damage to him. I knew right from the beginning, even before I was doing the Ninth Step, that he was on my list. So my main amends to him has been trying to be a different parent. I called him maybe two weeks ago and said I've been thinking about how we were. And I made an amends, and it wasn't received well by him, but still . . .

Her son was now drinking excessively and gambling.

> He said I don't want to blame you, but you never encouraged me to do things. He also feels that I took from him, because I went to a lot of meetings.

Inevitably, some amends are tied in with financial or legal complications, as addicted people are often not so scrupulous about these issues. The circumstances can be most awkward. You may recall Dan, the retired executive who attended church at times. His drinking was leading unavoidably to a breakup in his marriage, because the family had become increasingly disrupted. He described how this played out while he and his wife were on the verge of their divorce:

My wife and I were arguing over IRS issues, like trying to file back taxes and straighten out our lives, and she wouldn't give me the documents I needed. So I got some money and put it in the bank and used it to get the documents from her that she wouldn't release. She claimed I forged her signature, which I had. I was arrested for forgery, so I would not do my Eighth Step with her while I had this legal problem.

These episodes can certainly work out in idiosyncratic ways:

I settled things with my ex-wife in the court system; it got thrown out. I gave her the money she wanted and she gave me the documents. Then I did my Ninth Step with her.

The making of amends also can become embroiled in family conflicts that arose over many years. These conflicts may have lingered on if a resolution was not possible. For one patient, amends to his mother had worked quite well. ("I always knew you were a good boy.") His father, however, had himself stopped drinking, but the animosity between him and his son was longstanding.

My father didn't want to talk about it, because he never did his Eighth or Ninth Step with me. He said, "Listen son, you know what you do; I know what I did, so let's let it be." I was very frustrated with that. My sponsor said it wasn't my place to make my father uncomfortable. Fast forward a few years. My father was dying of cancer, and he asked me to be his health proxy. I was complaining to my sponsor about my siblings not helping out in the hospital visits with my mom. My sponsor reminded me of the Ninth Step. He said, "You know, maybe this is your Ninth Step."

Some hurts are resolved in unexpected ways.

A Perspective

Let's look broadly at the issue of resolving the misbehavior of the past. Conflict is inevitable between people, particularly when it is fueled by the poor judgment inherent in an addicted person's behavior. There has to be a way for such conflicts to be resolved. Ethologists tell us that this need is evident even in lower primates, perhaps giving us a perspective on how this is innate in human nature. Monkeys and apes can carry out a variety of behaviors that reduce stress between individuals to assure that prior aggression will not resume. Chimpanzees may kiss their former opponents after conflict.[17] Some monkeys may embrace or groom their former adversaries.

From the perspective of adaptive survival among social animals—people included—there is a need for ways to assure that a history of conflict does not rend the fabric of relations among close associates. People, of course, are more complicated than lower primates; they can reflect on the motivations and habits that generated the harm they have done to others, and the Bible distinguishes those who are righteous from those to whom amends are due: "Fools mock at making amends for sin, but goodwill is found among the upright" (Proverbs 14:9).

This is what it comes down to in a given AA member: In concert with her Higher Power she can strive to rectify her defects of character, but harm done to others cannot be that easily undone. What can an AA member then do in the face of this lingering debt? American culture embodies various themes on this count. A person designated as guilty can be relegated to social isolation. In this case, penance can be isolating and unproductive. In traditional cultures, ranging from early Christianity to religious practices among monastic orders, self-isolation and penitence could be practiced for actual or imagined sins. In the mid-nineteenth century, penitentiaries were developed where prisoners were kept isolated in single cells where they could reflect on their malfeasance (and do penance, presumably).[18]

Nowadays our seemingly more humane culture is oriented toward providing opportunities for rehabilitation within the society where harmful acts were committed. In terms of society overall, this can be carried out without punishment and by means of resolution, thereby avoiding justice by retribution. A more benign conception, though, is that of restorative justice, where repair of damage is the goal. The concept of a truth and reconciliation commission epitomizes this. In South Africa, the ills of apartheid could not be undone. The hope was that both the perpetrators and the victims could truthfully and openly describe what had happened, with the perpetrators requesting amnesty, so that an adequate resolution could be achieved without retribution in the form of punishment. This seems to have been surprisingly and fortunately successful in that case.

Intimate and close personal relationships are typically where AA members seek to make amends. As we have just seen, the success of such an attempt can be acknowledged if it relieves those who themselves have committed the offense. The amend is crafted by the sponsee, with her sponsor's help in framing just how to best approach the person she has harmed. If it is done to the satisfaction of the two actors, then the mission has been accomplished. But success measured by the reaction of the aggrieved person is harder to assure, and we have seen examples from "Sure, don't worry" to "I can't really forgive you."

Social psychologists have studied the responsiveness of romantic partners to apologies for hurtful acts they have experienced. An important contributor to success in these situations is the degree to which the apology reflects true empathy.[19] This may be hard to achieve when one is going through a list of the many people one has wronged. Often, one cannot summon up the empathy that might be helpful when one is uncomfortable in having to face those one has wronged. Nonetheless, the whole process of these Steps tends to refocus one on making changes in how one runs one's life. It is perpetuated, in effect, by the Tenth Step, "We continued to take personal inventory and when we were wrong promptly admitted it."

STEP ELEVEN: PRAYER AND MEDITATION

To be specific, this Step reads, "Sought through prayer and meditation to improve our conscious contact with God, *as we understood Him*, praying only for knowledge of His will for us and the power to carry that out."

In our studies of long-term AA members, we found that they experienced little or no craving for alcohol (or drugs), and when confronted with stress or drinking triggers they could pray to relieve their distress and avert the craving. The ongoing practice of prayer is part of the routine of long-standing AA members, and it can be practiced in many different ways. For some, it is routine: "I pray every morning and night, always." Or alternatively, "I don't pray to God in a regular way, but I do pray most days. The person who gets out of bed and gets on his knees annoys me." Later on in this book, we will be looking at the biology behind the effect of prayer, and "How It Changes the Brain," but let's now consider AA's view on this.

The Big Book explicitly includes two prayers members can recite: In Step Three, "God, I offer myself to Thee—to build with me and do with me as Thou will. . . ."[20] This addresses the intent of the Third Step, "to turn our will and our lives over to the care of God . . ." This injunction was lightened up in the AA book *Twelve Steps and Twelve Traditions*, indicating that, "The wording was, of course, quite optional so long as we expressed the idea."

A second prayer carries the message of Step Seven, wherein members ". . . ask Him to remove our shortcomings . . ." In line with that Step, the prayer includes, "I pray that you now remove from me every single defect of character which stands in the way of my usefulness to you. . . ."[21]

These prayers are not what most members recite on a daily basis. If anything, they are more likely to use the Serenity Prayer as a mantra. The Serenity Prayer was modified from earlier versions by the Christian theologian Reinhold Niebuhr[22] when he recited it in his church in 1947, and it is now often recited at AA meetings.

> God, grant me the serenity to accept the things I cannot change, the courage to change the things I can, and the wisdom to know the difference.

Although it has come to be associated with AA, the Serenity Prayer is often cited outside the program as sage advice; to soften a religious connotation, it may be read without the first word, "God."

Prayer may not come naturally to new members, although they are often encouraged to practice it, even early on. This difficulty is acknowledged in the AA literature: "We will remember how something deep inside us kept rebelling against the idea of bowing before any God."[23] For some, acquiring AA prayer practice works out well, even though they may have felt at a loss initially. Bonnie, a social worker, recalls such an experience many years before:

> I asked my sponsor a lot of questions in the beginning. How do I pray and meditate? What is it going to take me to learn? Do you sit on a mountain top and contemplate life or do I talk about my alcoholism to a tree? What eventually happened was that I decided to talk to God. I would be quiet in the morning and talk to God and have conversations with Him throughout the day. I still do this.

Bonnie is quite sane, married, and successful at her work, but her current experience with prayer bespeaks a relationship with her God that is almost conversational. At times of adversity God is there to accompany her, even communicating back.

> Sometimes you can say I get messages. I'll hear words or hear things. I don't know if I can describe it. Sometimes it happens that I have this voice in my head saying you are going to be OK. There are some moments when there are some challenges for me and I want to run away and hide and not deal with life. Then when I talk to God and ask for His help, a sense of peace comes over me. I feel it in my heart, and I hear that voice that says it is going to be all right.

Psychiatrists may be uneasy upon hearing people report occurrences like these, namely, that they are receiving messages or hearing words, but accounts such as these are not uncommon, and come from people who in no way seem pathologic.

The phrase that refers to praying "on our knees" was initially included in Step Eleven by the Akron AA branch, whose members were more oriented toward traditional Christianity. Nowadays, though, prayer can be broadly defined for some, even hardly described as a prayer as such, perhaps more allied with a relaxed, meditative experience. Karen, who, before she decided to go to rehab, used to party while her husband was at work, illustrated this:

> Every morning, unless I have to be somewhere, I get up early; I do some sort of physical exercise. Today, I took a yoga class at 8:00. And that was my prayer and meditation. I will go out walking. It's very beautiful here. We're surrounded by a vineyard; we're on the water. I watch the sunrise and I watch the sunsets. That is my prayer and meditation. Where I feel the closest to my Higher Power is out in nature.

Dan, who attends church with some regularity, made use of his religious background to employ prayer in dealing with the guilt he felt over conflicts with his wife.

> Sometimes it's relationship issues that I have to take responsibility for when my conscience is bothering me. I can't go to work the next day and ignore it. I talk to the God of my understanding and it helps me to do what I need to do. So my prayer and meditation helped me face up to what I had to do today, to give an apology to my wife. I had prayed to God for this.

For some, the opportunity to pray is a source of respite early on in their membership. When Laurel, the newspaper reporter, first became involved in the program, she was despairing and grasped onto prayer for consolation from God.

> When I first came in I had this sponsor. I was hanging out with women in AA, and really going to the meetings, and I did have conscious contact with God. I would go kind of meditative and go to a park and talk to him. I was praying in the morning and praying at night and even when I was going to work. We had a big bathroom at work and I would go into the bathroom and lock the door and there was a little couch, and I would sit on the couch and meditate, and that worked wonders. I haven't done that in years. Now it's more that I go to a meeting sometimes when I can and listen and share.

Laurel still keeps a stake in the relationship she established with her Higher Power, knowing she can call on it in time of need, but she has attenuated her active involvement in AA.

I think if I had an emergency, I would go back to re-visit my contact with God, and pray if I had to. You're not supposed to have a 911 God. That's really not how the program works, but I often think that that's what I would do.

This access to prayer in a time of need can indeed be a lifesaver of sorts. Here is how one woman benefited, though not necessarily by plan, and was rescued by the salvation her prayer offered:

When I was two and a half years sober, I was making amends to people I had harmed. I did a lot of dishonest things when I was drinking and hurt a tremendous amount of people. One of the people I went to, I told her what I had done. I owed her a lot of money, and I told her that I would pay her back. A couple of months later, I was at the store where I was working, and two people came up to my desk and told me I was under arrest. I had never been arrested before. The person I had made amends to had pressed charges against me. I knew it was a possibility, and they took me off to jail. I was there overnight. I didn't have my cell phone, so I couldn't call my sponsor. I didn't have my Big Book. I was working on my Eleventh Step, so I decided to pray and meditate. After that, it was like a sense of peace and freedom. I honestly felt like I was going to be OK. I had been hysterically crying for hours before.

The issue of prayer can be fraught with conflict for some members, particularly those who have difficulty fully accommodating themselves to the concept of God or a Higher Power. Prayers can then compound their problem. A patient of mine who had attended AA with regularity had this ambivalence about God and prayer, and because of it she always experienced some discomfort in the program. This was aggravated by the sponsor she had acquired and by attending her home group where commitment to God, allied with traditional religious experience, was pressed on members. This came to a head when her sponsor expected her to pray with her on the phone every morning. With some trepidation and fear of her sponsor's anger, she dropped her sponsor and switched to an AA group more compatible with her beliefs. But she never could really bring herself to pray.

A Perspective

William James defined prayer as "inward communion or conversation with the power recognized as divine."[24] For the established AA member, this communication is a regimen for maintaining the spiritual renewal that they see as central to their recovery. Each member arrives at his or her own way of praying, and each addresses a Higher Power that is endowed with the charisma of the fellowship.

Contact with one's Higher Power is, in the end, mystical in nature, and to quote James again, the mystical "defies expression . . . more like states of feeling than like states of intellect. No one can make clear to another who never had a certain feeling, in what the quality or worth of it consists."[25] If you take James's observation seriously, that prayer is imbued with an ineffable feeling, we can be left just talking around what an AA member's prayer actually is. At best we can say that it barely has been introduced with the few examples I have cited here. But we do want to make some sense of this mystical process, and to do this, the reader has to empathize to some degree with what prayer means to an AA member, even if she or he feels no connection with God or religious thinking. We need to enter into the realm of the person who prays with this mystical communication from the perspective of that person's experience.

Stephen Post is a scholar and minister with whom I have collaborated in trying to get an understanding of AA's spiritual nature. He related the AA ethos to what he called "the ontological generality" in describing how a person relates to the divine. He described this generality as located at the intersection of two axes: One is the human axis of love of both one's neighbor and one self; this is the personal and interpersonal axis. A second axis is love of God and God's love of self; this is the connection to God.[26]

One can imagine that the nexus of these two axes encompasses a God–self–fellow alcoholic intersection that we see in AA prayer: A member speaks with his Higher Power while embedded within the fold of other partners in the fellowship. This is because AA members as a group often do pray within the same fold, and their fellowship is bound together in their bond with a shared Higher Power. If you want to look at AA from a theological perspective, the intersection on the two axes bespeaks unity within the spirituality of AA.

Prayer is a common practice within the American public, although there is not necessarily the commonality of spirit that one sees in AA. One survey shows that 92% of people say they pray sometimes, and fully 65% say that they pray every day.[27] These figures clearly reflect diverse denominations represented differently in different parts of the country, but what the AA members hold in common is their sense of community. Their prayers, individually tailored, bind them together in their shared fellowship, strengthening their mutual ties.

Prayer can be characterized in various ways.[28] It can be directed inward to seek personal transformation,[29] and this is allied with the ongoing, lifetime personal inventory undertaken in Step Ten. It also can be directed outward, for carrying the message to other alcoholics (Step Twelve), or it can just involve asking for practical help. Finally, it can be directed upward, in seeking identification with God, expressing trust in Him and in being in His presence. All these can cover the diverse roles that prayer can play.

When a person is uncertain about what will befall them, they will ultimately have to attribute[29] a likely outcome to some actor, be it themselves, someone else, or just Lady Luck. But prayer provides comfort in the face of these uncertainties by attributing to one's Higher Power the meaning of events, even if they are adverse. That is to say, it relieves the distress of uncertainty for the person who prays by allowing them to feel that things will happen through God's will. Otherwise they would experience the tension of whether they themselves can control events.

Even the practice of psychiatry can be combined with prayer in the hands of true believers. We studied fundamentalist Christian psychiatrists[30] whose organization meets each year at the same time and city as the overall American Psychiatric Association. As part of our study, we polled them on what is the most effective treatment for various psychiatric disorders, as they would see it within their system of beliefs. They responded that the healing of certain mental ills like suicidal intent, grief reactions, and even sociopathy, is better done through Bible and prayer than by medications or therapy. (They did rate medications as more effective for schizophrenia and bipolar disorder.) Given the right cultural milieu, even professionals can believe that prayer can resolve the distress that might be ascribed to mental illness.

The comfort that long-term AA members get from prayer is evident in their experience of "God's presence," in their lives: For both the young members and the adult doctors we studied, some three-quarters reported that at the very least they "felt God's presence" on most days. What this apparently means is that for many long-term AA members, their connection with their Higher Power is embedded in their everyday experience, where God is with them in person in some way, often during prayer.

The psychiatrist Robert Coles found that having God as a real companion was common among many children, and as AA does in its literature, and much as we have done here, he drew on references from oral history. Rather than number-crunching empiricism, he relied on storytelling. In *The Spiritual Life of Children*,[31] he described how some children are confident that they hear God in their thoughts. For them at least, "God's presence" can be experienced as real. Perhaps this is a skill that is lost by young people as rationality impinges itself on them and they progress to adulthood.

But even adults can learn to converse with God and hear Him speaking back to them under the right circumstances. The anthropologist Tanya Luhrmann[32] joined the rather unique Vineyard Christian Fellowship in Chicago, and visited with them in their church and in their homes. She found that over time members were able to acquire the capacity to "hear" what they "knew" to be the voice of God. Each would learn how to identify thoughts and images as an actual interaction with God. This was a skill that they had to practice to perfect. She wrote about her encounter with members of that fellowship:

> But as I listened to people talk about God, and about the way they experienced themselves in prayer, I began to think that these faith practices and the way they taught people to pay attention to their minds and emotions shaped something about the process of mind itself and that these changes helped people to experience God as real.[33]

The long-term AA members can also deal with God's presence as real. Some accept it comfortably, almost passively:

> His power and spirit have entered me in that I am now neutral. This has entered me in a way that is always with me and always there. It becomes no question of me saying yes or no.

At times, some may feel his presence but may, to their regret, need to struggle to assure its continuity.

> To some extent I am always in his presence, but I also know that sometimes I also look away. If I don't engage, I may choose to do something that blocks my connection, and I may make bad choices. What do I do then that will bring me back in line and back in conscious contact with Him? Sometimes I weaken that connection, so what happens then?

For the fully engaged, prayer is an act that can reinforce a connection with a Higher Power. Clearly, though, it is a practice that is not consolidated without considerable commitment, and time spent in the program.

STEP TWELVE

Step 12 includes, ". . . we tried to carry this message to alcoholics . . .," underlining a key aspect of AA membership, namely, bolstering one's own recovery by helping others afflicted by the same illness. In the Big Book, after Bill W tells of his redemption and explains the AA program, a chapter is devoted to how to approach fellow alcoholics to encourage them to turn to the fellowship. Bill emphasized, and also told AA members to be clear on this, that helping another alcoholic "plays a vital part in your own recovery."[34]

"Carrying the message" is central to the established AA member's mission. On the most immediate level, it means telling a new attendee at a meeting to "just come back." But this does not mean forcing oneself on anyone; instead, one should rely on relating one's own story to the newcomer, in order to provide an understanding of how one found a path that the other person can follow. Bill learned this through failing in his early attempts at spreading the AA message, when he found that preaching and importuning did not engage other alcoholics to join with him.

Spreading the word need not always be a passive process, and there are times when a soul is saved by active intervention. Frank, a patient of mine, told of when he had a relapse after leaving rehab. He was drunk, wandering in the street, when he encountered fellow sober alcoholics from an AA group he had attended. He was all but stuporous. They took him back to his apartment and he fell into a dead sleep. When he awoke the next morning he was afraid that he had been robbed. Instead, he found that his room had been put in order, and dishes he had left in the kitchen sink had been washed and put away. He was always mistrustful of other people's help, but he later told me, "This wasn't what I expected from people. It left me touched." He never took another drink, and realized that the only way he could recompense what they had done for him was to do likewise for other alcoholics. He later played a major role in establishing a residence for sober addicted people.

AA members are always vulnerable to relapse and withdrawal from the group, because the idea that an alcoholic cannot have even one drink is counterintuitive. In this respect, the fellowship is a social system that is vulnerable to collapse from within, and in light of this, its emphasis on recruitment makes sense relative to assuring its stability. Acquiring new members has the effect of validating the fellowship's philosophy. The Twelve Step role, therefore, carries an implicit message: Because we can successfully induct others to our philosophy, our philosophy must have validity. So in addition to assuring growth rather than stagnation in the membership, the recruitment process also validates the faith of the members themselves.

The emphasis placed on "giving back" was made clear to me while I was at an international conference of Young People in AA. Some 5,000 registrants were in attendance at a hotel in New York, and one evening almost half of them were in the hotel ballroom, seated theatre style, when a speaker's charisma left everyone riveted to her inspiring talk. She told of how she would break into neighbors' houses as a young teen just to steal their liquor and nothing more, how her life moved from desperation to ruin, and how she had compromised her own children. Then she spoke of how she found redemption in AA, and was now raising the daughter of her sister who had not been as fortunate as she, and had died of a heroin overdose. The audience was captivated by her. But then she told them that it was for them to reach out to others suffering from addiction. Now that they were sober, this was the mission they were obliged to carry out. It was an injunction that was most compelling, and the logic of her presentation had left her and the audience clear on what their recovery should lead them to do.

AA's Eleventh Tradition came to be, "Our public relations policy is based on attraction rather than promotion . . ." Organizationally, however, AA seeks to set the stage for new members to be brought in. Local intergroup associations list meetings on their websites. They also have telephone hotlines that alcoholic people or their therapists can call for advice on which meetings would be best for them. Each locale has Committees for Professional Cooperation to make information available to people who treat alcoholics.

Intergroup will also schedule members to conduct AA meetings at local hospitals. When I set up our units for addicted mentally ill patients at Bellevue Hospital, we had the local AA intergroup provide members to run an AA meeting on the ward every night of the week. When I spoke with the members of Young People in AA about substance abusing youths on our adolescent psychiatry unit, they provided leaders for groups there, too. There was always someone to run these groups; if one day's leader was ill or had another commitment, a substitute would be supplied.

It is interesting to consider the economic value of these voluntary efforts. Healthcare costs for alcoholism in a recent year have been calculated at $230 billion.[35] Nonetheless, it is estimated that only 15% of people with alcohol abuse or alcoholism actually receive treatment.[36] Perhaps more to the point, as many as 25% to 40% of patients in general hospital beds (the higher figure would certainly apply to Bellevue) are being treated for complications of alcohol-related problems; these are the people most severely affected.[37] AA members, although hardly a medical treatment in themselves for people affected in this manner, do represent a resource committed to helping such alcoholic people. Given the AA willingness to carry the message, its members could no doubt be better utilized than they are now.

The sociologist Max Weber discussed charisma as a captivating talent and gift that is understood to derive from some divine or transcendent source.[38] A charismatic leader embodies this special power, and Bill W, by virtue of his "white light" visitation, his dedication, and his compelling words, illustrated this gift. But the influence of a charismatic leader over his followers can last only as long as he (or she) is there to bear influence. One way a group founded on the basis of a leader's charisma can survive and continue to be effective is for the charisma, in time, to be imparted to a bureaucracy to which the leader's authority is transferred. For a religious group, this can be a priesthood. For a political group, it can be a party structure. Let's consider how this applies to Bill W and AA. Who will be invested with "carrying the message?"

The charismatic role of Bill W (and Dr. Bob) was soon shared with an AA Board of Directors and its role, in turn, was passed on to the AA General Service Conference in 1951. Delegates were sent to the conference from the five thousand groups across the United States and Canada,[39] which had emerged by then. The conference and the board of directors, now called the General Service Board, framed Twelve Traditions, essentially a code of conduct for members.[40] The First Tradition pointed out that, "our common welfare comes first. But individual welfare follows close afterward," making clear that there needed to be mutuality and support among the groups, even if they are self-governed. It further made clear that, "Our relations with the general public should be characterized by personal anonymity;" no one gets to present themselves publicly as speaking for AA.

In 1962, the General Service Board published Twelve Concepts,[41] emphasizing that AA's message is framed by the "group conscience," as expressed by a system of elections, from the local group level up to the General Service Board itself. In addition, the Traditions also emphasized that the fellowship's operation would be "nonprofessional," and this assured that the charismatic zeal would remain unmodified by salaried regulatory bodies, and that no AA member merited a greater authority or charismatic role than another in spreading the AA philosophy. This is important because the role of helping others lies in the hands of members who are of equal status, whatever their cultural background or economic class. These latter developments, wisely conceived, many of them at the behest of Bill W, are central to how AA has been effective in maintaining continuity. It is in the fellowship's members that Bill W's charisma is invested.

AA needed to have a vehicle for spreading its word in print and articulating developments within the fellowship as they arose. *The Grapevine,* the international journal of the fellowship, fulfills this role. It was started by six volunteers in 1944, but was soon seen as a vehicle for unifying the widespread and diverse groups. Between 1944 and 1971, Bill W published some 150 articles[42] and editorials in *The Grapevine,* leaving a legacy of AA's culture and mode of operation, and passing on his charismatic role in this way as well.

Although communication with new members takes place through personal contact, a key feature of AA also rests in its many other publications, all prepared with approval of the General Service Conference and the Board. The Big Book, for example, is published in a remarkable array of languages, forty-five in all, from Afrikaans, on through Korean, to Zulu. Other books, like *Sober Living* and *Daily Reflections*, serve as additional resources for members. Published pamphlets convey specifics on the implicit rules of membership, from "Questions and Answers on Sponsorship" to "The AA Member—Medications and Other Drugs."

The zeal for carrying the message, that is, for bolstering AA as a functioning system, does have limits due to its nonprofessional nature, its code of anonymity, and an injunction against a sizeable operating budget. These limitations have been good for the fellowship in that they defuse the possibility of members' self-aggrandizement and pursuit of personal gain. Certain entities have arisen, however, to carry out AA's potential for expansiveness in ways that AA's formal structure cannot. A look at some of these is useful in gaining an understanding of AA's dependence on volunteerism and its sustained success.

On an individual level, members can carry out numerous roles as emissaries for the program while still protecting their anonymity. In rehabs and sober houses, residents with some time in Twelve Step-based abstinence can take on the task of bringing newly admitted people to community AA meetings. Recovering rehab staff can volunteer as well. AA group members do "service" in making coffee, serving as greeters, and taking on administrative responsibilities. And, of course, with a record of sobriety, members can serve as sponsors for new recruits.

Upon first opening up our Bellevue ward for the addicted mentally ill, we had hardly set up any of the new programs, such as activity therapy or social work groups. After a few days, however, two posters, each one measuring some two by three feet, one with the Twelve Steps and the other with Twelve Traditions, were already bound to the wall. Clearly, one of the recovering staff had taken this task upon himself.

When I began research, I relied on AA volunteers willing to participate. In conducting our studies, I had no idea of how well members might accept this intrusion into their recovery. Indeed, some—even members of the local Committee on Professional Cooperation—said that any collaborative effort with a professional or researcher ran contrary to the Traditions. Other AA members were willing to accept our research as ultimately useful for "carrying the message." With understanding and support they gave their time and effort for alcoholics who would someday need doctors' help to send them on to AA meetings. When we were conducting focus groups, members dedicated time to travel to our site to participate. Members also volunteered to participate in the (hardly pleasant) time spent in the MRI brain imaging machine for our neural study, which I describe later.

Physicians in AA recovery embody this zeal as well. In 1949, Doctors in Twelve Step recovery established a society, International Doctors in AA, which now counts approximately 4,500 members among its ranks.[43] Members have local meetings and an annual international meeting, and they are ready to help colleagues who suffer from addiction. A third of the doctors I studied at an AA retreat, who had an average of two years in recovery, were themselves dedicating considerable time to addiction treatment.[44]

Young People in AA is a collection of autonomous local groups dedicated to helping addicted adolescents and young adults. These groups are emerging in various locales around the country and overseas and provide information on the Internet regarding the availability of AA meetings where youths predominate. Their annual International Conference of Young People in AA, in its fifty-second iteration, was most recently held in Florida. Each year, based on a prior presentation with detailed planning, a site committee from a given locale is chosen for the next year's conference.

The Oxford House model, quite different from most residential rehabs, illustrates how AA was brought into a community setting without recourse to a professional superstructure. In 1975, a former Senate committee staff member who was in recovery had been living in a halfway house that closed down. Along with other residents of the house, he took over the facility to set up a program based on Twelve Step recovery. It operates with modest rental fees from its residents, who are expected to work to support their upkeep. Today there are more than a thousand Oxford Houses. Most Twelve Step meetings are conducted when residents themselves are not at work. The facility thereby combines engagement in employment with Twelve Step-based recovery. The communal residence has been said to embody the residents' Higher Power to some extent.

This community-based model has been adapted in other settings where dedicated leadership and community support are available. Dr. Charles Silberstein, who had been a fellow of mine, undertook one such project. He had directed our halfway house for addicted men at the Bellevue Shelter, and he now serves as the only psychiatrist living on Martha's Vineyard, an island off the coast of Massachusetts. He set up a residence where local addicts can live, participate in AA groups, and work in the community—all self-governed by the residents. Frank, whom I mentioned earlier, who was brought home by other alcoholics when they discovered him drunk, had played a role in establishing this residence after moving to the Vineyard, thereby "giving back."

CHAPTER 6
Sponsorship

What are sponsors supposed to do? They have no job description or even a job title in the Big Book, but one could say that they have three jobs in relation to their sponsees: telling their own stories, providing emotional support and practical advice, and encouraging the sponsee to work the program.[1] Working the program means going to meetings, "working" the Steps, and, ideally, doing some service. In doing this, sponsors are central to the continuity of AA as an organization. Without them, new members would go astray, and the Steps would be no more than a cumbersome process to be short-circuited, if attended to at all. Sponsors are key to the whole system.

But what is in it for the sponsors? Why would they devote hours of their time to newcomers whose experience is fraught with anxiety, rebelliousness and so frequently, with relapse? Frank Riessman,[2] a social psychologist, considered many examples of people volunteering to help others who have the same problems they do, AA being a prime example of this. He referenced a list of over two hundred groups in which people help others, and, in doing so, apparently benefit from their participation.[3] Riessman came up with the concept of the "Helper Therapy Principle." His point was that if we focus on the persons being helped, we actually miss out on where the most benefit is derived, that is, for the helpers themselves. He pointed to research[4] that showed that when people have to improve on a speech supporting a particular point of view, over time they tend to change their own attitude toward that very point of view. So in AA, the helpers get support for addressing their own problem, and acquire a greater commitment to the process they are putting forward.

Bill W came upon this very principle of helper therapy as he developed ways to "carry the message" to potential members. He makes this point in the Big Book in the chapter, "Working with Others," wherein he tells AA members how to address the drinking alcoholic:

> Outline the program of action, explaining how you made a self-appraisal, how you straightened out your past and why you are now endeavoring to be helpful to him. It is important for him to realize that your attempt to pass this on to him plays a vital part in your own recovery. Actually, he may be helping you more that you are helping him.[5]

This benefit is evidenced in the outcome of one large-scale federal study, which showed that helping other alcoholics and serving as a sponsor was more likely to yield a positive outcome than the number of meetings a member attended.[6] When we ourselves studied long-term abstinence among members, we found that serving as a sponsor predicted a person's likelihood of reporting no alcohol craving at all.

The helping principle shows up in diverse settings. One study on intravenous drug users in AA and NA found that being a sponsor, rather than having a sponsor, is what yielded an improved outcome.[7] A study of people in communal living residences like Oxford Houses also described the important role of helping others.[8] And interestingly, when elderly, non-alcoholic married couples were followed up over a five-year period, it was the individuals who were helpers, rather than the ones who were helped who experienced the most relief in their distress.[9] Even alcoholic Aborigines trained to help fellow alcoholics gained more benefit than those they helped.[10]

Active sponsor involvement can enhance the success of a Twelve Step program in an interesting way. The folks at the NA World Services Office report that after the United States, Iran is the country with the most NA groups. (NA's tabulations show that the United States has 26,397 groups and Iran has 16,793.) I met with NA's coordinator for Iran and tried to understand what was responsible for the fellowship's success there. Granted, Iran has a very big problem with heroin addiction,[11] but what makes for NA's effectiveness in Iran became clear as we discussed how sponsors operate there. They work closely with sponsees individually, but also get their sponsees together as a group, encouraging them to support each other and provide them practical help outside of the regular meetings, even for their families. This approach derives from the nature of social relations there. You can see that when a culture supports sponsors having such a role in the real-life aspects of the recovery of other addicted people, the program can thrive.

DIFFERENT EXPERIENCES

Working one's way over the course of AA membership can be intimidating, particularly for someone who is timid by nature. Bonnie had been afraid to walk into her first AA meeting, and she had to build up her self-confidence to accommodate herself to becoming a sponsee, and then ultimately to sponsoring others. She recounted how she initially solicited a sponsor, and how she moved on from there:

> I needed someone in my life that I could at least talk to. I have to say I was intimidated by her at first. When I finally got around to asking, I was so nervous and afraid that she would reject me. But then she knew everything that I could possibly go through. For five years I called her every single day. I told her how my day was and what meetings I went to. She heard all of my crying, ranting, and raving, and also my laughing. She was my rock. After five years, she told me she didn't think I needed to call every day anymore.

Although the time seemed appropriate, Bonnie was frightened at the prospect of becoming a sponsor herself. As she described it:

> When I became a sponsor, my ego got the better of me. I went into a panic. I went back to my sponsor and told her I picked up a sponsee who had situations in her life that I couldn't help her with. After a time, if I didn't call [my sponsee] back, she would get annoyed. I prayed for help to get to the point where I could tell her I couldn't help her with certain things. She was going through marital problems, and I have never been married. I had to bring it back to the focus of AA when she drifted into other areas. She needed a lot of my time. . . . I have grown up in AA now. I am not as needy as I used to be.

One approach to sponsors' solutions for their sponsees' difficult problems is to resort to advising them, "Go to more meetings." This can be supportive, or it can ring hollow. AA members, though, when they go to a meeting feeling troubled, usually leave feeling better. At other times, however, such advice simply means that the sponsor has no answer for resolving the other person's life problems.

Finding the right sponsor is not always a straightforward process. What evolves depends on the character of both the sponsor and the sponsee,

and their needs and expectations at various points in the recovery process. A successful relationship is generally well structured, with clear
expectations for abstinence and for working the Steps. But there are as
many scenarios of sponsorship as there are AA members.

Arnold, a successful executive, had an uneven path moving toward
recovery, one that reflected the relationships he had with various sponsors. As a teen and young adult, he had been a rebellious drug abuser
and womanizer; rebelling, he explained, against his experience with an
oppressive and controlling mother. He was now married to a woman in
long-term recovery who pressed him to go to AA to deal with his drinking,
because alcohol was now compromising life at home with both her and
their two teenage children.

His first sponsor "was a hands-off kind of guy" who had developed a
small social circle of recovering alcoholics who got together weekly after
their home group meeting. Some in the circle were his sponsees, others
were just AA acquaintances. As Arnold recounted about the sponsor, "He
liked talking about women a lot. . . . I was content to glide along." And he
did glide along for a time, enjoying the company of the program members,
and staying sober. His sponsor defined no regimen for him other than not
drinking, and expressed no expectation of his working the Steps. At one
point the sponsor moved away, the group disbanded, and Arnold relapsed
to drinking.

Arnold went back to AA some months later. His second sponsor was
younger than him, less successful in business, and somewhat in awe of
him. As time went on, Arnold began drinking, did not tell his sponsor,
and eventually let the contact between them taper off. He then relapsed,
drinking heavily, and it was only after another year, under pressure from
his wife, that he decided, as he said, to "undertake the program seriously."
He started going to meetings on a daily basis, went into therapy, and
turned for sponsorship to a fellow AA member with whom he had been
friendly. Almost from the outset, however, a problem arose between them.
Arnold did not like being told what to do, and said that the sponsor

> . . . went from being a normal guy to acting like a Nazi. I didn't call him for a
> day, and he got on the phone and called me up and started yelling at me . . .
> I was out of town for a week or two, and I got a text saying, "Where the hell are
> you?" I said I know you think I should call every day, but what are you so angry
> about? . . . He didn't want to listen to me.

Arnold dropped this sponsor, but said that they remained friends and
still socialized at meetings. Being earnest about maintaining his sobriety,

however, Arnold promptly decided to acquire a new sponsor. He chose someone whom he saw as congenial, with whom he felt comfortable, and began working the Steps. The two got along well and, "He understands enough not to take my bullshit. He can hear it; he can read it; and he'll tell me about it." Arnold finally achieved stability in the program.

As a teenager, Jared had dedicated his considerable intelligence and engaging nature to getting into trouble rather than to applying himself to his college courses. Jared, too, switched sponsors, but without relapsing. By age twenty-two, he had been to rehab, having abused multiple drugs, dealt some cocaine, and then became addicted to narcotic pills. He came out of rehab, entered therapy, and began going to meetings, making sure not to resume contact with a girlfriend with whom his relationship had been laced with cocaine and pills. He missed her sorely, nonetheless. After two weeks, upset over the loss of his girlfriend, he purchased some Percocets (narcotic pills) from a dealer he knew. He took a few at once, and then realized the downward course he was risking, and got scared.

> And that very day, I went to a meeting and ended up sitting next to someone that I had seen at meetings before. I was so upset, and asked him to be my sponsor. There was no other reason at the time other than I was in a lot of pain mentally.

The new sponsor took him out for coffee at a local diner. He had a circle of AA friends, ones who were supportive of Jared's recovery. They were a good deal older than he, and he seemed to thrive in their company.

Jared, who was multiply-addicted to pain-killers and cocaine, had come from an affluent family, and was now returning to school at a local college to finish up his degree. He said that the social class difference between him and the others—they were from working class backgrounds—did not present a problem in their relating with each other. Sponsors are often of a different social class than their sponsees, but their program-based relationship can supersede other issues.

Jared was, however, concerned that the relationship between him and his sponsor was less formal than he had wanted, and after a few months he turned to another person in the group of members he had connected with to serve as his sponsor.

> We called him Vegas Bob. Every day of his life was about AA. He was kind of a floater, he worked at Dunkin' Donuts sometimes, and sometimes he worked at a sports memorabilia store. He was my sponsor for a year or two. He taught me

about being humble and grateful for life and for the things I have. I would go to meetings with him every day. I was lucky he had so much time on his hands. . . . He was there when I needed someone to hold my hand. I remember sitting in the diner with him and crying about how my life was over because I could never get my old girlfriend back.

By the time Jared was completing college and beginning to work in his father's accounting firm, he turned to another sponsor for a year, one who encouraged him to do service in the program and speak at institutional meetings in local hospitals. (Jared's rather engaging personality was helpful in his becoming an articulate advocate for AA.) Another sponsor whom he finally took up with, and continued to see over the years, gave him the structure he was seeking:

He is extremely disciplined. He gets up at 5:00 in the morning, meditates for a half hour, has the same structure every day. That's what I needed in my life these past years.

As we can see, sponsors can fulfill different roles along the course of one's recovery. If a member is committed to sobriety and the relationship is constructive, after a time, movement from one sponsor to another can work out well. For those who achieve sobriety and move on from AA and then still stay sober, a sponsor for that limited time of active membership can be quite useful. Being in therapy with a professional who has experience in addiction treatment can be invaluable in helping someone as they move from one sponsor to another, as it was for both Arnold and Jared.

Karen illustrates another aspect of a sponsees' experience, namely, how some members stay committed to one sponsor over many years. During her earlier, wayward years, Karen partied on cocaine until she had to sign herself into rehab, having realized that she was falling deep into addiction and compromising her children. She was now sober for fifteen years, and had moved with her husband to a rustic exurban area. She still kept up with her sponsor as a resource to help her reflect on difficult issues that might arise:

I don't call her very often. I call her when I'm really in a spot and need to vent. I call her if I'm really, really unhappy. I call her if I have a question and I'm not sure how to handle something. On a rare occasion, I will call her if I have a question about a sponsee.

I always get right to the point with her, and then I'll say that's where I'm at. She'll say something to me like, "You know Karen, these people that pass through your life, they're only here for such a short time. You're putting too much energy into this. Why are you worrying so much about it? Before you know it, they'll be out of your life." At first I'll get mad. Then I think about what she says, and then I'll figure it out on my own.

If the fit is right, and if the sponsor can be judicious and provide useful reflection or advice, relationships with sponsors can persist long after a sponsee has worked the Steps. In such cases, sponsors can help a person, even one reasonably well adapted, to deal with difficult situations from time to time. When I asked Karen if her relationship with her sponsor was different from therapy, she said:

It's not different from therapy. The difference is she's my sponsor. I'm not paying her and she knows me really well. She's been my sponsor for years.

The term "therapeutic alliance" is used to characterize an abiding and trusting relationship between patient and therapist premised on a mutual commitment to the patient's needs. A good alliance is thought to be key to successful therapy. What Karen has described about her relationship with her sponsor reflects this very thing. Knowing that her sponsor is there for her, and then being able to respond positively to the sponsor's supportive statements, makes for a meaningful source of assistance in a time of need. This, in fact, is key to a good therapeutic alliance. The fact that her sponsor is not a paid professional does not detract from the "therapeutic" value of this relationship. Wouldst that all patients had such trusting relationships with psychiatrists or psychologists they go to see.

Karen is a woman who is mentally intact. Many who come to AA, however, are suffering from appreciable mental illness, as well as needing support in addiction recovery. For the more dedicated members of AA, sponsoring a mentally ill person presents its own challenges, which should include encouraging the sponsee to get professional help. Mentally ill chemical abusers (MICAs) can present problems for a sponsor. These can include knowing how such sponsees should be supported, especially those who have ambivalence about taking their medications. This latter problem is sometimes heightened by what some members describe (erroneously) as an AA philosophy that recovery is only valid without medications that affect one's feelings. One member described how some of these issues can play out:

A sponsee of mine had suffered a psychotic break, so I visited him in the hospital and encouraged him to work with his doctors. He is still a member of AA and is sober, and he still has work to do, as we all do. He doesn't like being on medication because he heard that you're not sober when you're on meds, and maybe he does like the buzz that he gets when he is manic. I encourage him to take his meds.

He will ask me to tell him what to do from time to time. I don't like to tell him how to do things, but rather I help him be responsible for his decisions. He is almost invariably at odds with the world. I'm not going to tell him he is right all the time. I just try to be a bit moderate with him. Most people won't put up with a sponsee like this.

Another member describes how these problems can exceed what she can handle:

I had one MICA patient who would call up and rant and I would just hang up, so she would call me back and apologize. She had a bad experience when she was a young girl, a lot of trauma. She fixated on this and on earlier experiences. I pressed her to go to the doctor and to take her medication, but she wouldn't, so I told her I couldn't continue as her sponsor.

LAY THERAPISTS

If Karen saw her sponsor as a therapist of sorts, and some sponsors try to help their MICA sponsees maintain equanimity, one might wonder: Have lay therapists, ones without professional training, been found to be effective? In fact, is there a need for unschooled people to treat those with the broad variety of psychiatric disorders (including alcoholism)? We can safely say that there certainly is a gap between the need of the psychiatrically ill for stable treatment and what is actually available. The best data we have on deficits in treatment for the seriously mentally ill derive from a major national survey conducted by the federal government. It found 6% of the population to qualify as seriously mentally ill, but less than 40% of them were receiving stable treatment.[12] For alcoholism, the gap in needed care is even worse. The World Health Organization reviewed cross-national epidemiologic studies and found that 73% of people with alcohol abuse and dependence in the United States go untreated.[13] So absent a flood of new professionals, it would be good to have something constructive to fill this gap.

We can trace nonprofessional community care for the mentally ill as far back as the thirteenth century, to a unique tradition in the city of Geel, Belgium. In Geel, mentally ill people could spend their nights in the local infirmary and go out into the community during daylight hours to be cared for and even work with the local populace.[14] Until the twentieth century, however, when help became available for alcoholics, such assistance was pretty much up to local churches and preachers.

There is only a modest literature on lay therapists' place in settings where professionals might otherwise operate. Mothers who were at high risk for parenting difficulties have been counseled by lay community members in one program; this was shown to be of benefit on some issues like providing social support, but not on others, like resolving family conflicts.[15] In one British program, lay therapists were given the role of facilitating cognitive behavioral groups for anger management. Although initially daunting for them, this was seen as positive overall.[16] This is certainly an issue in less industrialized settings. In Goa, India, the effectiveness of primary care clinics in caring for patients who were designated as having "mental disorders" was improved when lay counselors were added to improve on the professional services.[17]

Two controlled studies carried out in the United States yielded interesting results in this regard. In one, the outcome of treatment conducted by female college students who applied to run therapy groups for hospitalized schizophrenic patients was compared with the outcome of psychiatrists and social workers who conducted similar groups. On certain tests of performance designed to distinguish normal from psychotic people, the college students' patients actually did better than those who were in groups conducted by the professionals.[18] The best that the research team who conducted this study could do to explain their results was to "conjecture" that the college students' "naive enthusiasm" and use of "less stereotyped" activities might have contributed to their better outcome.

Perhaps the most telling of such studies was carried out by Hans Strupp,[19] a highly regarded psychotherapy researcher at Vanderbilt University. He assigned male college students suffering from "depression, anxiety, and social introversion" to either professional therapists with "a reputation in the professional and academic community for clinical expertise" or to college professors without such training but with "a reputation for warmth, trustworthiness, and interest in students." Sessions were conducted twice weekly for four months. On average, no difference was found between patient outcomes.

What can we learn from all this? It may not be surprising that the enthusiasm and commitment for AA that characterizes AA sponsors can be effective. Interestingly, though, it has been found that the benefits of sponsorship regarding maintaining sobriety are derived early on in spon-sees' affiliation with AA, rather than later on.[20] It may be that in the early stages, sponsors' investment is most needed for providing support, a model for identification, and—as Jerome Frank famously pointed out[21]—hope for recovery, the key ingredient in any psychotherapy.

CHAPTER 7
Spiritual Awakening

After completing the first eleven Steps, AA members are ready for the final one, which begins with the phrase "Having had a spiritual awakening. . . ." Step Twelve is not included casually. It harkens back to a seminal moment in the genesis of the fellowship, an episode that members refer to as Bill W's "white light experience." In December 1934, Bill W was admitted to the Towns Hospital on the Upper West Side of Manhattan for a fourth episode of drying out. He was despairing of hope at that point, but later wrote of a transformative experience he had while there: "It seemed to me, in my mind's eye, that I was on a mountain and that a wind not of air but of spirit was blowing."[1]

This was a spiritual awakening for Bill, dramatic in quality, and one that would serve as a model for future AA members seeking redemption from their addiction. Even today, generations later, there remains an expectation of transformation that serves as a turning point in members' own recovery. For some it is sudden and dramatic, and for others it comes on more gradually. Nonetheless, most long-term abstinent members who have made peace with the need for abstinence can recount having had some such experience, albeit typically much less dramatic than Bill's.

I became particularly attentive to the importance of this experience after reading a study carried out by Lee Kaskutas and her collaborators,[2] who followed up alcoholic people after they had been discharged from treatment. The respondents who reported having had a spiritual awakening at some time after discharge were almost four times more likely than others to achieve a stable abstinence. Given the reports I had heard of such awakenings from AA members, and along with this striking finding, it seemed important to research such experiences in a systematic way.

Was there support for such research? Spirituality and belief in God are not, to say the least, topics on which the U.S. federal government focuses its research support. In fact, some years before, I had been asked to participate in a panel at the National Institute of Mental Health (NIMH) to discuss the psychology of new religious movements. There was a small protest by members of one cultic group, which had apparently had gotten wind of this. The NIMH dropped the whole venture summarily. "Church and state" remained separated. The John Templeton Foundation, though, was more recently open to research related to spirituality and religion, and I received funding to embark with my colleagues on a series of studies on various subgroups of the recovering Twelve-Step community. We embedded this issue in the surveys that we employed.

One result in particular was most interesting: We had framed the studies to measure the impact of spiritual awakening on Twelve Step members' addictions, and in the midst of a longer survey we asked participants to rate the degree of craving for alcohol or drugs they had experienced in the previous week on a scale from zero (not at all) to 10 (extreme). Later in the survey, they were asked to indicate whether or not they had experienced a spiritual awakening. We surveyed attendees at a conference of doctors in AA, most with long-term sobriety; 81% reported having had a spiritual awakening. Those who reported affirmatively on this were twice as likely to have experienced no craving at all in the previous week than those who reported no such experience.[3] Results were similar for younger members at an international conference on AA. A large majority of those surveyed indicated that they had had a spiritual awakening, and those who had were again most likely to experience no craving at all.[4] In addition, I had a working relationship with the central office of Narcotics Anonymous, and they cooperated in a nationally grounded survey of their members. The results there were equally compelling.[5]

If one thinks about it, addicted people coming to experience no craving at all is remarkable, given that alcohol and drug addiction are characterized by a craving that drives people to relapse. In fact, the latest psychiatric diagnostic manual (DSM V) includes craving as one of the criteria for diagnosing addiction. Additionally, when one treats people who are in early recovery, it becomes clear that for many of them a compelling craving for alcohol or drugs is a key factor in their difficulty in maintaining abstinence. They may describe this as an ongoing pressure or they may be compelled to seek out a drink or call a cocaine dealer based on a pressing impulse.

I also began interviewing numerous AA and NA members of long standing about this in the hope of getting a feeling for just what spiritual awakening was, and whether one could generalize across long-standing members to see what characteristics, background, and experience they might have in common.

We should begin, though, by looking at how AA itself describes the issues of spirituality and spiritual awakening in the Big Book:

> The terms "spiritual experience" and "spiritual awakening" are used many times in this book which, upon careful reading, shows that the personality change sufficient to bring about recovery from alcoholism has manifested itself among us in many different forms . . . Most of our experiences are what the psychologist William James calls the "educational variety" because they develop slowly over a period of time.

The members' stories varied greatly, describing intensely personal reactions and differences in when, where, and how awakenings took place. Each account, however, bespoke a deeply felt transformation.

FEELING JESUS'S PRESENCE

An awakening can be very dramatic in character, as reported by Ben, a surgeon who had worked long years in our municipal hospital system and had retired on a pension, while living alone and unmarried. He had occasionally drunk too much before retirement, but once his daily responsibilities were gone, things changed. He reported that

> I was in my mid-fifties, an alcoholic, a pothead, a sex addict. Something had taken over me and I became obsessed with the clarity that cocaine seemed to offer. I wanted to get high, and that became my value in life. It came to the point that I couldn't do simple things like pay my rent, and I was always on the edge. I didn't think how I could ever manage money again.

By that time Ben had not worked for three years; he had been arrested once for a DWI, and two times for possession. Now he told how his recovery began:

> A stranger showed up while I was buying crack: he gave me an offer I couldn't refuse, and I went to rehab. It wasn't that I didn't know I had a problem, but I just didn't think there was any release. I was there in rehab with 50 bucks hidden in my sock. I wanted to get out and get on a subway and come home.
>
> I went outside the building and was having a cigarette, when all of a sudden a sense of peace came over me and I didn't see it, but I felt the presence of

a person, and in my mind that person was Jesus. It was strange. I was sort of embarrassed. I felt his presence, and then a peace for no more than three or four minutes. This seemed to be part of a message. I was set to come in from the cold. And then I listened and let these people help me. I realized that it was not about judging, it was about acceptance.

Afterwards, I didn't really talk about it. I left out the Jesus part. Now, even when I am in a shitty mood, it comes out and I have a moral compass. It's a spiritual tool that continues to impact me. It gets richer and leaves me less depressed, less isolated, and less upset with what's wrong with me.

Ben's experience was dramatic and sudden, and took place early in the course of his recovery, in fact, before he had gotten a grip on the concept of how abstinence could be part of his life. Like many addicts first encountering AA's pressure for abstinence, he had hoped to "cheat" the consensus he confronted. He had money in his sock and a plan to take the subway back to his source of cocaine. In the context of an awakening, however, God, as it were, caught up with him in the form of the presence of Jesus and summoned him to accept what the folks at the rehab center were offering.

FINDING GOD AGAIN

Many AA members have come from families where religion was accepted as a matter of course. Over time they became disillusioned regarding any belief in the existence of God or in the validity of religious practice, only to later find Him in the course of their awakening. As Janet, a social worker, described it:

I was an atheist before AA. I had been religious and went to religious school when I was young. I had a very alcoholic family, every kind of violence and abuse. I had asked God to change a couple of things when I was eleven and he didn't, so I concluded there was no God. I wasn't just an atheist but an angry atheist. I invited Jesus freaks into my house when they knocked on my door. I questioned them for hours just for fun.

Early on in the program I stood in my living room one night and said, "I don't believe You are up there but if You are, get off my fucking back. You do everything for everyone else, but nothing for me."

Before I did the Third Step ["to turn our will and our lives over to the care of God"], I said, "I don't really quite believe that you are there, but I hear that I have to do this to stay sober. I don't believe that I have to give you my life but I will give you that car outside. God, I offer you my old Chevy," and I read the rest of a prayer. The car got totaled within the next couple of days. I was not in it. No one understood how it happened. I got more money than if I had sold it myself. I went to the meeting that night and got a sponsor.

Later on my sponsor made me do the Third Step on my knees, in a church. I wouldn't have done it two months earlier, but I was willing to do whatever she said. That night at the AA meeting, they were talking about honesty. I thought I was honest, but by the time it got around to me in the short hour, something changed. The words that came out of my mouth were, "I'm a worthless piece of shit." Twenty minutes before the meeting I would have told you that I had a little problem with drinking. I didn't realize that I had lied, cheated, connived, and then fast within the meeting I realized I had. I knew what the Jesus freaks meant when they said they were reborn. I had experienced it.

The transformation that Janet underwent is typical of many members. During her collapse into addiction, she concluded that her traditional religious background, and God as well, had failed her. Her recovery then took place in the form of a generic acceptance of AA's "God *as we understood him*," a benign and caring figure. This was fueled by a coincidence of events, the totaling of her car. At least in retrospect, she perceived this as a signal of the coming of redemption, ascribing the event to a word from above. This attribution of coincidence to a higher power is not uncommon among members, and serves as evidence of the hand of God operating in one's life.

Janet's feelings of worthlessness laid the groundwork for a coming redemption. Like an errant sinner, she got on her knees and effectively sought forgiveness from a higher power—all this fueling the redemptive experience of her spiritual awakening. Her prayer, as in Step Eleven, was a powerful tool for ritualizing commitment to the fellowship program and protecting against the impulse to drink.

AN OUTSTRETCHED HAND

We can consider another phrase from the Twelfth Step, "we tried to carry this message to alcoholics. . . ." This phrase has great meaning for members. Lending a hand to another alcoholic person to help pull them out of the chasm of their drinking is as lofty a goal as an AA member can have. It also served as a turning point for this fireman, two and a half years sober:

I can say that God could do for me what I couldn't do for myself. Not by trying to fill me up as an empty vessel, but to make the purpose of my day bringing joy to others. I would never have believed this. Once I did this I was able to get rid of want and need.

I didn't get into doing service until I was about eighteen months sober. I committed to a four-hour telephone shift at intergroup. When I did that, it was an out of body experience. It was the first time in my life that I did something without looking for anything, and that's when the bells went off and I've never wanted a drink since. I was going to meetings every day. I did the Steps, but I hadn't had the service, the selflessness, the unconditional love.

The experience of "carrying the message" in and of itself served as the basis for an awakening for this man, who realized he had been isolated and self-involved beforehand.

The experience of empathy conveyed by another alcoholic can be transformative. Years of addiction can leave a person with a profound loneliness fueled by their having compromised many close relationships, and then having felt isolated and rejected by their family and friends. On the other hand, people coming to AA meetings are accepted unconditionally, and find themselves immersed in a culture where they are potentially no longer alone. This inevitably has an impact on them if they can stay on, but it may take time, particularly when their own commitment to abstinence has not been firmly established: "How can I honestly feel accepted if I'm not fully in keeping with the expectation of other members?"

A symbolic act of friendship and acceptance, as one woman experienced it, was able to turn all this around, particularly when it came from someone with whom she could identify:

When I kept hearing the sobriety stuff that people were talking about, I knew that in my alcoholic family the drinking would lead to death. So I leaned toward the sober path they were recommending. But I never had what you could describe as a spiritual experience. I was blocked off from the world and didn't connect with people . . .

I used to follow a woman out of the AA meeting and just nod to her. She was sober for eight years. I wouldn't go to coffee with her because I thought she was too busy. I did this for months. One day, I was afraid to go home because there was a lot of wine in my house. All I knew was that I found myself delaying her at the street just to actually say hello. Then she said, "You are really lonely aren't you?" All of a sudden it was a watershed. She really understood; she knew what it was like for me to be a drunk. The pilot light of my soul hadn't been extinguished yet, and she detected it. It was really recognizing that I wasn't alone; I had a soul that was worth saving. I got to AA with the 1% of me that wanted to live and that was the spark of soul that I still had, and AA helped with the other 99%.

A GRADUAL REALIZATION

For many members, a spiritual awakening is neither sudden nor dramatic. It can be an ongoing and continuing process, but no less meaningful than if experienced with great drama. Here is how one woman described a more gradual experience when I asked her about an spiritual awakening:

> I was a functional alcoholic for a long time, but about three or four years in, I was no longer functional. I was trying to stop and I couldn't. That's when I called AA. Now when I think about it, I got this enormous sense of relief of being with people like me and knowing it was possible to not drink. I thought my story was horrendous, but I heard other people and found that their stories were really bad, too. Then one day I was walking along the beach in Nantucket and it was 5:00 PM, and I realized that I didn't have the compulsion to run home and have a drink, and it was a great relief. I go to AA every morning at 6:30 AM and see the sunrise, so every morning I have a spiritual experience. That's my spiritual experience. They're not big epiphanies but, along the way, little 'ephiphanets.'

The expectation of having a spiritual awakening leads people to interpret their experiences as reflecting an awakening, even if they do not experience it dramatically. They may even have been told by another member that their awakening had taken place. Here is how one person explained this:

> So I heard about it from meetings and in The Big Book, but I couldn't identify with it and didn't really know what it was. I was thinking that I should have had a spiritual awakening by now. I was questioning whether I was an alcoholic. Then it was gradual. It wasn't a trumpets blaring, angels singing moment for me. My sponsor was the kind of guy that would whack me in the head with the Big Book. He told me, "You had a spiritual awakening. You are sober. You aren't craving the drugs," and I thought about it and realized that. My sponsor told me that I had had one and guided me in the direction to understand that I had one.

A SURVEY

I wanted to see if we could develop a systematic understanding of the experiences people affixed to their awakenings: For whom did these come about in a sudden manner, and for whom did they emerge more gradually, over time? Was it common for people to have a sensory experience, something like that which Ben, the retired surgeon, had while standing outside the rehab building? Did they take place in the midst of adversity, as in the depths of drinking?

To answer questions like these, I turned again to the doctors' group of longtime AA members, and they agreed to have their members surveyed again at one of their conferences, this time about spiritual awakenings. Given that many of them may have had more than one experience of spiritual awakening, we asked them to describe what their first one was like. The majority reported that it had come about gradually rather than suddenly, and took place while they were working the Steps rather than before or afterwards. Almost half had used alcohol or drugs the week before, but less than one in ten the week thereafter. The majority reported that they had experienced a craving for alcohol the week before their awakening, whereas only half that number felt that in the week after. The depression they experienced declined materially as well.

Given that awakenings presumably put people closer to their higher power, could this be measured? The majority of those who had an awakening reported that they now felt God's presence in their lives on a daily basis, but only a minority (less than one in seven) of those who had not experienced an awakening felt this way.

Altogether, we documented a diverse group of transformative experiences, ones that did indeed bolster the doctors' commitment. In many respects, however, the uniqueness of such experiences is most compelling. To my mind, the various experiences members described are what most illuminated the process. The awakenings are personal, and illustrate the individuality among respective members.

A PSYCHOLOGICAL PERSPECTIVE

The drama of these experiences is often so personal and compelling that one is reluctant to look for generalities. For a scientifically minded psychiatrist, though, it is hard not to seek out some psychological principle that can shed light on an underlying process. In doing this, it would be hard to apply the kind of biological model that predominates in psychiatry nowadays; this model is adrift in a sea of chemical reactions that take place both within neurons and at their interfaces. It is employed to direct attention to chemical changes that may explain why people are depressed or anxious, and then to pharmaceuticals that may resolve this. The same model can be applied to addiction, peering into the brains of addicted people by using techniques like functional Magnetic Resonance Imaging (fMRI) to spot what goes on in their world of neurotransmitters, and in various brain areas. But we are not about to catch people like Ben or Janet at the moment of their awakening, rush them into a laboratory, and check out what is transpiring in their brains. We might even miss what is going on in their minds; that is to say, the thinking and feeling that they themselves would describe may be more relevant anyway.

Another approach can be drawn from behavioral psychology. It relies on promoting gradual changes in the way addicted people on the way to alcoholism fall prey to the triggers that lead them to drink excessively. The alcoholic is encouraged to consider all the circumstances that make him want to drink, and all the places that are associated with his drinking, in a setting of cognitive behavioral therapy. This technique is certainly helpful in psychotherapy, and is typically part of a process of learning how to avoid relapse. It does not, however, capture the dramatic transformation that is evident in the descriptions of those who experience a spiritual awakening.

The kind of transformation that I have described taking place when people were inducted into cultic movements seems pertinent here. At some point during the course of engagement into AA, a tension emerges between two views that a given person may hold. These are:

(1) the recruit's accepting abstinence through faith in a higher power, and
(2) the recruit's alcoholic identity as someone who thinks that at some point they could drink again.

The way this tension between two conflicting beliefs is resolved can help to explain why a dramatic awakening may take place.

Here is some background: In the 1950s the psychologist Leon Festinger[4] saw an interesting opportunity to study a doomsday cult whose members believed that a flood would destroy the world on a particular day. In advance of the expected cataclysm, many members were telling friends and family of their fear, and were even giving up their property. Festinger saw this as an opportunity to find out what happens when people are accepting two conflicting thoughts that are incompatible. In the case of this doomsday cult, it was their "knowledge" that the world was ending and their observation, when that designated day came, that the world would (presumably) not come to an end. He and his research team joined with the cult members to see what these believers would come up with at that time.

The cult members were confronted by the tension between the two seeming realities: anticipated destruction and the evidence no such event was taking place. Festinger termed this conflict of perceived realities, "cognitive dissonance."[5] The cult members had to develop some explanation that would resolve the conflict. Their leader provided this by claiming that the world had been spared because of the "force of good and light." The cult members' attitude was rapidly transformed, they readily accepted the explanation, and began spreading the cult's new belief[5] even more diligently.

How does this conception of cognitive dissonance apply to a spiritual awakening in AA? The paradigm runs like this:

(1) A belief is held with deep conviction: "As an alcoholic, I believe that I can resume drinking at some point."
(2) A contradiction arises that runs counter to it: "I have joined AA as an alcoholic who cannot ever drink again."
(3) The dissonance: "I can drink" vs. "I can't drink."
(4) A resolution now comes about: "I'm seeing that this contradiction is resolved by my Higher Power because I am now spiritually awakened."
(5) This way of resolving the dissonance is supported by other believers. "I see that other AA members who are supporting me say that they, too, have had a spiritual awakening, so I should, too."

The AA literature and long-term members have set the stage for this way of resolving the dissonance by means of a spiritual awakening.

There is a demand characteristic of being a member, that is to say, there is an expectation of a spiritual awakening experience built into the culture of group membership. This demand characteristic frames the way the resolution of the cognitive dissonance is subjectively experienced, as an intense feeling of realization and enlightenment.

This resolution of cognitive dissonance pertained to the disenchanted youths I studied who responded to many of the new religious movements of the 1970s, and who were unhappy and open to a new outlook on life. It is an age-old type of experience seen in religious conversions historically. In our Western culture it dates back to St. Paul, who as a zealous Pharisee persecuted the followers of Jesus. On the road to Damascus, as a light from heaven flashed around him, Jesus appeared to him, and he converted. All are primed to attribute their circumstances to a new perspective and to "flip," as it were, their attitudes toward a new experience, and thereby find relief from their distress. This relief is experienced as a new, "enlightened," and positive state of mind of the awakened self.

In AA, uncertainties and distress have been alleviated by accepting belief in a higher power guiding one's life. The process may seem mysterious, but if it is implicit in a subculture, as it is here, where participants are primed for dramatic change, it is indeed dramatic change that may well befall them. Reading the Big Book text and hearing speakers at meetings contributes to the expectation for such change and can become a basis for how an awakening is achieved. Clearly we have begun to gain a perspective on awakenings, one that begs for further elaboration, given that we do have a long way to go in understanding such a dramatic event.

CHAPTER 8

Further Involvement

Regular meetings listed on AA websites demonstrate a local AA community's focus on committment to its members, but the worldwide Twelve Step fellowship itself also defines a community of closely held relationships of a more global and abstract nature. This global fellowship image is much like a devout Catholic's inclination to see the worldwide Church as vital to him, as much as is his own parish. The sense of having ties to a broader community reflects a sense of belonging that in many ways has been lost in contemporary society. The idea of this loss is underlined by authors like Robert Putnam in his influential book, *Bowling Alone*,[1] in which he documents the decline over recent decades in civic organizations, clubs, even bowling leagues. In many ways, AA addresses this need for community.

We found this in our study[2] of both new religious movements and of the AA members themselves. The response to measures of feelings of affiliation toward their movements overall was as strong as feelings of affiliation toward the individual, local members they knew best. Ties to a universal community carry great meaning for people. This is made all the more meaningful when, for example, they attend their local parish church. Here they are part of a larger whole.

This shows up in AA, with extended Twelve Step activities beyond the local groups. They range from holiday parties for teens and young adult members, to retreats for older folks, to AA-related affinity organizations, to cruises for sober people. I would like to describe some of these to show how some members' lives can become involved in AA beyond the established meeting structure. These activities enlarge the AA universe for those who participate, but are independent of the AA General Service

Office. Because of this, the people involved do not have to comply with AA traditions like maintaining anonymity; they can keep membership lists. They can also deal openly with a variety of drugs, even overeating, smoking, and the like, not just alcohol.

Young People in AA is an example of a network of members, many of them relatively new to the program, who have organized themselves with remarkable effectiveness. Early on, they started having annual conferences—efficiently run, heavily attended, and replete with great enthusiasm. These conclaves have now been held each year over recent decades, each time in a different city, and each conference sponsored by a local network of young AA members. The conferences are remarkably well organized, run entirely by volunteers, and require only a small registration fee to cover the meeting site expenses.

As I have mentioned, we did one of our AA studies in cooperation with the International Conference of Young People in AA in New York. Over 4,900 people were registered to attend, and my staff and I were allowed to set up tables near the conference registration site to enroll participants for our survey. Many AA meetings and discussion groups were held over the course of the three days, and the enthusiasm of participants and the camaraderie of people of diverse social backgrounds and nationalities reflected the remarkable reach of the network to youthful alcohol and drug addicts worldwide. Most of the smaller meetings there were run along the lines of the typical AA meeting format, and some were dedicated to particular subgroups, like Spanish or French speakers, or gays and lesbians. At one meeting that I sat in on, a young woman from Norway spoke of a near miracle: that someone else had been prepared to attend, couldn't go, and instead underwrote her flight. She had come without a place to stay, and was put up in the hotel room of another attendee she met at the airport.

At one session, some two thousand young people sat quietly, theater-style, as a middle-aged woman, clearly experienced at speaking in an inspirational way, gave a talk. The next evening's program included a dance with very loud music and hundreds of young people celebrating. There was neither a drink nor any rowdy behavior evident at the whole conference. And remember, these were kids whose collapse into alcohol and other drug problems was so bad that they needed to go to Twelve Step meetings almost daily. This came out clearly in our survey. International YPAA now has a website where, as of this writing, over 400 groups worldwide are listed. Most are in the United States, but there is representation in twelve other countries, too.

Internet-based contacts are another network phenomenon. They have now generated other large networks of Twelve Step members of any age, who can stay in touch with one another no matter where they live. One example of this is the website, *In the Rooms*, established by two men in Florida in long-term recovery. With over 300,000 registered members, it offers extensive addict-related information, and effectively provides help for people to maintain their sobriety. Among its resources are weekly Skype-based Twelve Step meetings. Some AA members apparently find these video meetings to be helpful for staying sober, although we have no research-based experience to show the benefit they might provide.

Destination-based retreats are an integral part of many spiritual and religious communities; their purpose is to deepen participants' experience and understanding of their faith. In a sense, AA's retreats have a similar function, to immerse participants deeply into the spirit of the fellowship. They typically extend over the course of a weekend and are held in a secluded or rustic setting. Participants eat together, hear inspirational talks together, and participate in break-out discussion groups.

Although AA is not a religion, this does not mean that it is not likely to develop retreats for its dedicated members. The fellowship is based on a belief that relief from suffering is achieved through acceptance of a Higher Power. In this respect, it is not surprising that it has developed retreats like those of some religious denominations. To carry this analogy to religious retreats a step further, a given AA retreat may be sanctified, as it were, by association with a figure considered to offer a revered symbolic meaning in AA's culture or history.

The Matt Talbot retreats are carried out by organized groups, defined by members who live in respective locales, like a town or a county. Like regular AA groups, each Matt Talbot group is independent. Inspiration for them is heightened by their association with the spirit of Matt Talbot, an alcoholic dock worker who lived most of his life with his mother in Ireland at the turn of the twentieth century. One evening, penniless, and with no credit left to get drunk at a local tavern, he decided to "take the pledge" to renounce drinking. The pledge was something that alcoholics would do in Ireland at that time to become abstinent, often for a month or two, but Talbot stayed sober for the rest of his life. He might have gone unnoticed by history, were it not for the cords and chains discovered on his body when he died suddenly. In 1972 he was declared as "venerable" by the Vatican, meaning that he had the personal qualities to become a saint.

Another group sponsoring retreats, "Came To Believe," owes its inspiration to Clarence Snyder, a sponsee of Dr. Bob, the cofounder of AA. Snyder's story appeared in the first versions of the Big Book, and his sponsees developed the retreat format with locations in both the United States and Great Britain. Here is how one retreat in Florida was announced in London. It was held in August, hardly the Florida tourist season.

Discover the "Why" and "How" of our AA, CA, NA, OA, Al-Anon Programmes. Clarence Snyder, one of the first 40 of AA. He helped to write the "Big Book" and founded the "Came to Believe" spiritual retreat in Florida USA to give alcoholics and their families an opportunity to enjoy a life-changing experience. "How long do you want to be sick?" Clarence used to say. "The Steps are like a medicine capsule with *12 ingredients*, you take them when you want to get well!"

Although regular weekly AA meetings represent the core activities of the fellowship, YPAA and retreats such as these suggest that other options can develop around regular meetings, some related to specific subcultures. One example of this are the Grupos de Quatro y Quinto Passos (Fourth and Fifth Step Groups).[3] These first arose in Mexico, and have since been established in sizable numbers in States with large Mexican émigré populations. Entry into the program begins with an intense three-day retreat, after which participants attend a group meeting almost every night of the week, where they are promptly offered sponsors as guides. Although the Grupos use the Twelve Steps of AA, they strongly emphasize the Fourth and Fifth Steps, which relate to soul-searching and, in this case, giving intense testimonials that "go deep" to "let it out." These may relate to personal matters, like depression or prior sexual abuse. It remains to be seen whether, in time, a splinter program like the Grupos can stay fully within the AA fold, and be listed by the fellowship on its websites.

Here is a thought. How will the AA membership numbers go in the future? Who will attract new recruits? Let's consider the three groups we have just discussed. The retreats are conducted for people who are committed to the fellowship and sustain the attendees' zealous involvement, but their focus is not on enlisting a new generation of members. The Grupos members will pass the word on to the Mexican American community and may provide a variant of AA to this expanding segment of the American population. YPAA's people, on the other hand, represent an important segment of the fellowship's future within the broader population, as is evident in their remarkable conferences.

Those in our contemporary society who are most unclear about their mission in life may be found among a generation of adolescents and young adults who are just emerging from the envelope of their nuclear families and their parents' value systems. Because they have yet to gain a sense of what is meaningful for them, many turn to alcohol and drugs to fill the gap where a sense of purpose would otherwise be lodged. It is hard to know how many of these youths will fall over the cliff of recreational drug use down to a level where a fellowship like AA is needed, but let us consider

Jack, and the commitment to the program's future he has acquired. We discussed before how he was failing out of college when he encountered AA. He is now a personable twenty-seven-year-old lawyer who had achieved sobriety in AA. Jack was one of the organizers of New York's Young People's conference. When we asked for help, he arranged for us to set up our study there, and he later recruited subjects for our AA brain-scanning study. At Young People's AA meetings, he helps people to connect with sponsors. As he said,

> Once someone gets sober as young as I did, and has been as involved in YPAA as I have been, you have a lifetime of street cred. Even now that I'm older, I can go to young people meetings, do service-related stuff, and be accepted as one of the gang. . . . My main title, in the Queens [New York] YPAA is secretary, and I do a ton of things under that. I'm YPAA's representative to the Queens County General Service, so I'm sort of the point person between them and YPAA. And I'm also the current chair of our ad hoc digital communication guidelines subcommittee.

It is not necessary to have a lot of young people who have committed themselves the way Jack has to keep addicted youths moving into the fellowship. It is people like him who will do whatever they can to "carry the message" to a generation of new members.

PART III

Alcoholics Anonymous in the Setting of Addiction Treatment

CHAPTER 9

Its Place in Medicine

It is appealing to consider doctors as scientist-clinicians, applying what is presumably the product of peer-reviewed research with technical finesse. But in reality, most of the treatments applied in day-to-day medical practice have not been subjected to the rigorous standards of scientific research, and most have not been studied under controlled conditions. This means that clinicians are practicing more of a craft than a science when they intuitively apply the skills they have learned, hoping that their best efforts will relieve their patients of suffering. Much of their work is, therefore, based on their experience and on the judgment they exercise in difficult clinical situations.

The treatment of alcohol and drugs clearly falls into the domain of "difficult clinical situations." Each patient's motives and social circumstances are particular to that individual. In treating addiction, doctors face a situation in which they are far from having scientific solutions, or even mutually agreed-upon treatments, for most aspects of this disease. How does AA fit into this somewhat murky domain?

When I entered the addiction field in the 1970s there was little alternative for doctors to support their alcoholic patients other than referral to AA. Over these last decades, a variety of psychotherapeutic approaches and medications have been developed that are helpful in treating the alcoholic, but for many of the most severely afflicted, AA may, in effect, be their only ticket for assuring survival. Nowadays, though, there are questions as to whether insurance companies will reimburse patients for treatment that is based on an AA-oriented approach. Certainly, payment for residential rehab facilities, mostly Twelve-Step-oriented, is usually not supported by insurers, even though the most severely compromised people may have no other recourse.

Contemporary medicine aspires to apply the model of logical positivism, a nineteenth century philosophy of research developed around the physical sciences. This scientific perspective posits that what cannot be measured does not belong in the domain of science. It is easy for biochemical models and even physically bound medical problems to be judged by this standard. Given this, it has seemed reasonable for academic physicians to dismiss AA, which arises out of a spiritual experience, as falling outside the domain of their armamentarium. AA has not helped with this. It has contributed to making it hard to measure how well it works by separating itself from the professional and research communities and maintaining the anonymity of its members. Furthermore, medical research tends to shy away from the kind of psychological mechanisms that underlie the fellowship's operation. Nonetheless, given AA's value as a resource for addicted people, often one of last resort, it is important to develop an understanding of its role in the medical system.

AA has never been subjected to controlled studies because of its Traditions. One consequence of this is evident in a report of an early analysis of AA-related medical literature,[1] which includes only randomized controlled trials. It concluded that "there is a lack of experimental evidence on the effectiveness of AA," or that "AA helps patients to accept therapy and does not keep patients in therapy any more or less than other interventions." For those researchers and physicians who have misgivings about AA, this report is often cited as evidence that AA does not match up to the standards of contemporary medicine, and it has even been cited to imply that AA does not represent a valid approach for helping addicted people.

More recently, a number of controlled studies have shown the effectiveness of AA. One analyzed results of a large-scale federal study on alcoholism treatment where the results of AA-facilitated treatment were measured.[2] Another was on an interesting approach to introducing patients to AA in a group therapy approach.[3] These have taken into account the difficulties in randomization. It turned out that this group induction, in the hands of professionals, was quite well received by staff in a number of treatment programs. In fact, when I visited Israel, where alcoholics, and hence AA sponsors, are hard to come by, one counselor had been using his therapy group for alcoholics as an ad hoc sponsoring session. Our own studies have also shown how AA already has helped many people who are in Twelve-Step-based recovery, but of necessity, we could not randomize them to contrast them with other alcoholic people who did not attend AA.

Because of the AA tradition of nonaffiliation, at best, it stands side by side with medical care. AA can hold meetings in hospitals, and patients can go to community-based meetings, but these stand separate from ongoing medical functions. They are, in effect, a voluntary adjunct to ongoing treatment. The fellowship does, however, have a history of positive relationships with certain members of the medical community, and this goes back to its very beginning.

Doctors were certainly involved in the emergence of AA. Rowland Hazard was a successful investment banker who needed expert help with his alcoholism. In 1926 he traveled to Zurich, Switzerland to seek out Carl Jung, a psychiatrist and leader in the development of the psychoanalytic movement. When Jung found that he could not help Rowland with his own brand of treatment, he told him that his only hope was to achieve a spiritual awakening or a religious experience, which might repair the spiritual deficit that Jung felt was inherent in the compulsion to drink. On returning to the States, Rowland spoke to a friend about his experience with Jung, which was instrumental in helping Bill W move his own spiritual awakening toward collaboration with other alcoholics. In 1961, Bill wrote to Jung to express appreciation for his help with the patient Rowland Hazard. He also expressed appreciation for Jung's writings, which were read by many AA members. Jung replied respectfully. His letter included the classic phrase, *spiritus contra spiritum*, spirituality provides a recourse from the ravages of alcoholic spirits.

Another physician played a role for Bill W, helping move the transcendent experience he had in the Town Hospital in 1934 toward a constructive end. After his "white light" vision, Bill thought he might be "crazy," but William Silkworth, the medical director of the hospital, told him that his experience was not the result of a mental aberration, nor was it a hallucination, but rather, a spiritual breakthrough. Silkworth, who believed alcoholism to be a biological "allergy,"[4] later invited AA members to help with the patients in his hospital.

And then there is the physician cofounder of AA: The fellowship is considered to have been initiated some months after Bill's spiritual experience while he was struggling to stave off the desire to drink while in Akron, Ohio on a business trip. In order to be helped, he was introduced to a physician, later called Dr. Bob in the AA literature, who also was struggling to deal with his alcoholism. They spent days together trying to understand their illness and stay sober. Bob had one more relapse to drinking the following summer but remained sober thereafter. The encounter between these two men, a layman and a physician, led to it being said that any two alcoholics who struggle to help each other with sobriety can constitute an AA meeting.

Dr. Harry Thiebout, a psychiatrist and director of a sanitarium where he treated alcoholics, was impressed when he came across the first edition of the book, *Alcoholics Anonymous*. He gave the book to a woman patient of his who, after reading it, came to be transformed, and was the first woman member of AA. In time, Thiebout undertook getting Bill invited to give a presentation at the Medical Society of New York, and in 1949, to the conference of the American Psychiatric Association (APA). This led to an important validation of the fellowship for doctors when Thiebout promoted the publication of Bill's talk in the APA's scientific journal.

DEVELOPMENT OF MEDICAL INVOLVEMENT

Harry Thiebout's introduction of Bill W to the American Psychiatric Association in the 1940s planted seeds for acknowledging the importance of AA in aiding recovery. Another key development had taken place in 1956, when the American Medical Association designated alcoholism a disease. By implication, AA was addressing a problem that had a legitimate place among the illnesses that doctors were obliged to treat.

Here is where things stood for alcoholism by the late 1960s. My own experience in relation to addiction medicine illustrates the way this field would emerge, and with it medical attention to AA. As a resident-in-training in psychiatry, I had been on night duty at our psychiatric emergency service, which consisted at the time of no more than one resident in an interviewing room, with pink "continuation sheets" on which to keep a relatively brief record. I remember a young man, who was in the throes of alcoholism, coming in and asking for help with his problem. As a scion of the best in psychiatry of that time, I told him that he had come to the wrong place, and suggested that he might get help somewhere else in the hospital.

But we can go back to 1973 to see how AA, and addiction treatment, began to find their way into the medical mainstream. The U.S. government was about to establish its national institutes on drug abuse and on alcoholism. It also had just developed a program for certain medical faculty to enter a Career Teacher Program to develop medical training in the addiction field, a program I was invited to join. This program had been seen as essential because medical schools at the time were virtually devoid of any systematic programs directed at this major public health problem, and certainly had none on the nature of AA and how it promoted abstinence among its members. Clearly, concepts like spirituality and spiritual awakening in the fellowship had not been systematically studied or taught. At that time, many doctors, even those few who were in the addiction field, had little understanding of the fellowship a half-century after it was founded.

My medical school was typical of training centers nationally, which were essentially devoid of faculty involved in addiction treatment or research, but my good fortune was that there was a small group of physicians in the alcoholism field, who were members of a New York City Medical Society of Alcoholism. As one of its founding members wrote, the Society consisted of doctors who, because of the nature of the patients they treated, "yearned for identity and legitimacy."[5] Because its monthly meetings were only a subway ride away from my office, I was able to meet its founding members. They were more than happy to see a young medical faculty member enter their field.

Dr. Frank Seixas of the New York Society came to meet with me, a junior faculty member in that same hospital. He took me down to the medical emergency service where an alcoholic patient was sick with the consequences of his disease. Seixas doted on the man, expressing concern for his plight and spoke with staff—all of whom had been ignoring the man—to assure that he got the help he needed. Given his expression of compassion, it became clear to me that alcoholic people, even those displaying the foolishness of their descent into drunkenness, deserved the thoughtfulness and concern accorded any other medically ill patient. This was not part of established medical training at that time.

Over time, I became active in that Society, whose members "yearned for identity and legitimacy." They were physicians dedicated to making the benefits of AA, along with whatever additional help they could provide, available to their patients. In time, they came to attract other doctors from around the country, and their society later was renamed the American Society of Addiction Medicine (ASAM).

Among its members were a number of doctors who were themselves in recovery from addiction. Douglas Talbott had been a respected physician, and a consultant to the NASA Space Program, before he collapsed into severe alcoholism, actually ending up on the street, to be saved by one of the early Society members. Talbott later played a role in setting up treatment programs for colleagues who were addicted. As a principal leader among them, he established a residential program for addicted physicians in Atlanta, Georgia.

In many ways Talbott epitomized the zeal for Twelve Step recovery that was so prominent among of clinicians who cared for addicted people at that time. He was eager to help out with any research undertaking I might propose, and allowed me to come to a biennial retreat in Atlanta for physicians who had graduated from his treatment program. While there, I was able to sit in on a Twelve Step meeting of the returning doctors. It had an atmosphere of profound commitment and solemnity, more so than at the few AA meetings I previously had attended in the New York area. It was most impressive how physicians could come to be such devoted AA members.

Around that time, I had become aware of an example of how group participation influenced people's thinking and behavior. This derived from studying contemporary religious cultic movements of that time. It helped shed light on how people also could be transformed through Twelve Step participation. All this later devolved into a research-based model for how AA could be presented to doctors in the addiction field to show that valid psychological principles bore on the fellowship.

Talbott and I had agreed that I could administer a survey to the attendees at the retreat (with their prior consent), one which would draw on similar ones I had used for the cultic youth movements.[6] The doctors' responses showed them to have a level of commitment to AA ideology as strong as that of the youths who had become affiliated with their own movements. Additionally, the doctors reported a level of improved mood upon joining AA, as had the youths when they had become engaged. This lent weight to the fact that there was a measurable process underlying these dramatic transformations. Among the recovering doctors, identification with the task of helping other alcoholics was intense as well. A quarter of those attending the meeting had even undertaken full-time careers in treating addicted physicians. The encounter with these physicians in recovery illustrated how one might work with the medical community around the issue of AA, by developing a research orientation for studying the fellowship.

Over the ensuing years, the struggle to get organized medicine to recognize addiction treatment as a priority was gradually succeeding. Medical services for addicts were being established in many teaching hospitals across the country. My own chance to develop a service arose on moving to the New York University (NYU) Medical Center, and its main teaching facility, Bellevue Hospital. Bellevue, located next to the East River in Manhattan, has the largest psychiatric service of any general hospital in America, and was the principal place where many homeless and mentally ill New Yorkers could turn for protection from their demons. Although it was devoid of addiction services for the many patients in its psychiatric beds, there was a growing recognition that substance abuse was playing a role in bringing about those admissions. Along with two fellow trainees who had come with me to NYU, we set up special units for people with combined substance abuse and general psychiatric disorders, like schizophrenia and manic depressive illness. AA, having eschewed professionalism and financially based treatment, could not operate in the services we set up, but it was apparent that there was a need for having Twelve Step meetings available to the patients in our service. I was able to bring in AA members to run meetings on our ward, but they had to operate independent of the medical hierarchy, in line with their traditions.

As time went on, it became apparent how important the Twelve Step experience was to many of our patients, but as often as not, this issue was not brought up by the medical staff taking their histories. There were many examples of this deficiency, as became clear in case conferences for the addiction psychiatry fellows I was training. One patient, severely depressed, bereft of any resources, and removed from family ties was living homeless on the streets. After he was admitted to our psychiatry service, as I wrote earlier in the book, I interviewed him at a case conference for my fellows, and he spoke of the many times he had considered ending his life. When I asked him why he had not done so, he said that he knew that he was always welcome at AA meetings for the homeless at a church near Times Square. For many AA members this might not have been surprising, but for us it was a lesson in how the fellowship offered hope for survival to our most damaged patients.

In ministering to our indigent patients, we emphasized the benefits of medical care, welfare payments, and the modest comforts of our hospital facilities, but the spiritual support of AA also seemed important to them. In order to see what the patients actually felt to be most relevant to their recovery, I had two of my fellows carry out a study. We had our addicted, mentally ill patients rank various offerings that ranged from professional help and creature comforts to opportunities for spiritual renewal and expressing belief in God. We used the same list for medical students and nurses, and later even for addiction psychiatrists, to see what they thought was most important to the patients. The results came through very clearly.[7,8] The patients ranked the spiritually oriented items the highest in terms of what was important to their recovery. The students, nurses, and psychiatrists ranked them lowest. Apparently, we professionals were not attuned to the importance of what AA offered and what could motivate our unhappy patients, compromised by substance abuse as they were.

This mismatch between what would inspire these patients to struggle toward recovery and what the medical community was inclined to emphasize was pervasive among physicians in the addiction field across the country, and it was inherent in the addiction training programs that were being developed for a generation of physicians to address the needs of these patients. In fact, the Society dealing with addiction medicine, which had lent credence to the importance of AA in its earlier years, was now moving toward an approach based on pharmacology, seeking out any medications that could be used for our patients. Most of these treatments (except for methadone, and later buprenorphine, for heroin addiction) were of little avail.

There was a need to bring AA more to the forefront in this medical community. I undertook doing this by working with a few highly astute colleagues who themselves were in recovery, setting up workshops at the Society's annual meetings. At the same time, our faculty at Bellevue developed training materials that could be used for medical educators to introduce their students to the value of spirituality and Twelve Step approaches for recovery. There was a reasonable hearing for this work, but it did not carry the same credibility as systematic research, which was the basis for credibility in the medical community.

DOCTORS IN TWELVE STEP RECOVERY

Most states have programs to oversee addicted physicians who are working to achieve a recovery. These programs are organized to help them while at the same time monitoring the quality of their practices. These doctors' progress is followed by staff to assure that they can return to practice medicine in a reliable manner. As it happens, they provided a setting for developing further research-based approaches to AA. The Director of the National Institute on Alcohol Abuse and Alcoholism knew of my research on Talbott's Virginia program, and on the strength of his recommendation, I was given permission to study doctors who were being monitored in the New York State physician's recovery program.

Almost all of the state-based physician monitoring and recovery programs were built on a Twelve-Step-oriented model. There were reasons for this, because they had to maintain a strong orientation toward absolute abstinence. If previously addicted physicians were to emerge while drinking occasionally or using cocaine if only infrequently, their reliability in managing patient care would justifiably be open to question. Furthermore, many of the physicians who were active in initiating these programs were experienced in treating patients with the Twelve Step format, and many of them were in recovery on that very basis themselves.

Our study of the New York State program provided opportunity to gain further understanding of how AA could relate to the medical community. Physicians under its supervision had been addicted to a variety of drugs, primarily alcohol and opioids, but also cocaine and benzodiazepines (like Valium). When physicians were reported to the program, they had the option of participating, but were told that if they did not, their cases might be referred to governmental authorities, with the possibility that they could lose their licenses.

After they were evaluated, they were treated and followed up by counselors to assure they were maintaining abstinence, keeping up competent workplace performance, and attending Twelve Step meetings. We found that a large majority of the physicians, among a series of records we reviewed, had indeed attended Twelve Step meetings with regularity. A small number of the entire group were at first reluctant to go, but had ultimately participated successfully in Twelve Step programs.

The issue of addicted physicians and their recovery through Twelve Step membership provided the means for us to get the attention of the medical addiction community. Research psychologists had carried out worthwhile studies on the outcome of treatment based on Twelve Step models. They had set up sophisticated approaches to finding correlates of recovery in these patients, but this work was getting little hearing among physicians. On the other hand, doctors could identify with the plight of their own colleagues who were suffering from an illness.

Some doctors in the American Society of Addiction Medicine were quite comfortable acknowledging that they were in AA-based recovery, and they set up their own AA meetings at the Society's annual convention. This was particularly true for the doctors who undertook working with their addicted peers. Others were still wary of the stigma that might be associated with this. One colleague of mine confided his story of recovery to me, but only revealed it openly to colleagues in the Society years later. He was a highly accomplished research professor in the addiction field. Not without justification, he had feared it might leave some of his research colleagues skeptical about his work.

One exception to this reticence stood out very clearly in the person of Dr. Don Kurth, who served as President of the American Society of Addiction Medicine. He was willing to tell his story to the members of the Society, to give them a source of inspiration for Twelve-Step-based recovery. He recounted how he had grown up in a middle-class family in New Jersey, but had begun hanging out with a group of substance abusing youths as a teenager and got addicted to heroin. Things went downhill rapidly for him, and by the time he was in his late teens he was essentially homeless, sleeping at times in a bus terminal in upper Manhattan. He ended up at a drug-free therapeutic treatment facility, and some eighteen months later emerged with a solid sense of the abstinence he needed to maintain.

Don had never applied himself at school, but decided at this point that he would try to enroll in a college near his family home in New Jersey. Given his prior record, he had to tell the Dean of his own recovery, and was rebuffed as an unreliable candidate for admission. After dejectedly walking out of the Dean's office, Don decided to turn around and present his case as assertively as he could, and did finally succeed in gaining admission. He told me he had no idea of how to study, given his marginal high school experience, but he went to the library and took out books on how to deal with classwork. He did amazingly well; he ended up being admitted to Columbia University's medical school, and from there he went on to a residency at Johns Hopkins. His subsequent career had been interrupted by a lapse into alcoholism, a bout at a rehab facility, and a return to successful practice. By the time he had joined ASAM, he had been a committed AA member for many years. His experience served as a vivid example for members of the Society of how AA can help the afflicted.

After a time, I was able to establish committees on Twelve Step recovery in ASAM and The American Academy of Addiction Psychiatry, both of the national medical organizations focusing on addiction in which I had played a leading role (as president). We developed position papers to be adopted in both organizations to support the promotion of medical education and research around the Twelve Step model to gain acceptance of AA as important in the organizations. We continued, as well, to run workshops for members and bring in researchers from other disciplines to present their findings to our conferences.

Our published findings brought the issue of Twelve Step recovery more to the fore in the medical community, but the actual experience of physicians in AA was compelling in itself to members of the societies. Many members were unfamiliar with the format of AA meetings as they had never gone to any of them as observers, despite the fact that this is an approach that AA welcomes. Videotaped interviews of AA members in recovery describing their experiences had a material impact on the doctors. A number of the workshops that we conducted at conferences included physicians in recovery who carried out model AA meetings for other members. Their stories were compelling to their colleagues.

There are, however, complicated crosscurrents in addiction treatment that impinge on AA's place in clinical practice. One influence that determines the way doctors view addiction treatment is the economic support behind research, which comes primarily from the two institutes within the National Institutes of Health that deal with addictive disorders, one for alcoholism and the other for drug abuse. Their combined annual budgets of $1.5 billion cast the die for university-based researchers who rely on this support to carry out their studies. But these two institutes are only a minority of the twenty-seven that constitute the NIH. The others fund studies on a myriad of illnesses, from cancer to heart disease to infections, and the NIH culture focuses heavily on biological mechanisms for developing new medications. This culture sets the standard for the institutes dealing with addiction too, leaving them primarily oriented toward research on biochemical treatments. Laboratory-based researchers do not get enthusiastic about the value of a fellowship that turns to "God as we understood Him."

A second major influence is that of the pharmaceutical industry. This is where revenue derives from implementing new treatments, and this is where researchers turn for drawing on support for patient-based studies in their wards and clinics. Some of this funding has yielded drugs with a moderate impact on alcohol use. Naltrexone was given an initial impetus for promotion by its licensed manufacturer, under the brand name Revia. An injectable long-acting form of it, Vivitrol, has been approved for alcoholism treatment as well. The National Institute on Drug Abuse has underwritten numerous studies on the use of medications for cocaine addiction that alter neurotransmission, or for developing a vaccine against cocaine, actually to little effect. Both of these factors, the NIH culture and the orientation towards pharmaceuticals, ultimately devolve into less emphasis on AA, a socially and culturally based option. It is not that the biological research is not valuable, but that it tends to move the addiction treatment culture away from needed attention to Twelve Step recovery.

One telling example of actual success in the medical pharmaceutical domain is the introduction of buprenorphine, which can be used for treating addiction to pain killers (as well as heroin). We can now examine how the painkiller problem came about and how it relates to the use of Twelve-Step-based treatment. The abuse of short-acting opioids has been a major public health issue for some time, as illustrated by addiction to drugs like oxycodone. With the introduction of a sustained release oxycodone preparation, OxyContin, its manufacturer undertook a major initiative to promote its wide use for pain. The manufacturer ran conferences and touted it as having only a modest risk of addiction (a claim that people expert in such medications could have reason to doubt). Excessive, even casual prescribing ensued, leading to addiction patterns that became almost pandemic. Sales grew from \$48 million in 1996 to \$1.1 billion in 2000.[9] By 2004, it had become the leading drug of abuse in the United States.

In 2000, buprenorphine was approved for the treatment of opioid addiction, based on federal research and on promotion by the pharmaceutical company that had patented it. Research on drugs for addiction treatment generally has not been profitable for pharma companies. Because of the denial of illness, addict patients tend not to take their medicine. Buprenorphine, however, is an addictive drug itself and as such people are likely to take it at least for a period of time. Because of this, it can be used in treating chronic opioid addiction, particularly because it is available from private doctors who are certified to prescribe it. (I am one of them.)

What impact did this treatment innovation have on the relationship between the medical community and AA? In fact, about one million people in the United States are currently being treated with buprenorphine. An assumption was embodied in the year 2000 legislation, namely that buprenorphine prescribers would be experienced in the treatment of addiction and would provide patients with access to supportive recovery-oriented treatment. In one study, relapse after twelve weeks of buprenorphine maintenance was nearly universal (92%).[10] In practice, little attention has been paid to providing any psychosocial support, AA included. The original limitation on the number of patients that an individual practitioner could maintain on buprenorphine was increased from thirty to one hundred. Prescribing buprenorphine with little to no attention to anything but the medication itself, a lucrative option for many prescribers, has become the norm for the large numbers of patients on this medication. In fact, many prescribers had little or no experience in treating addiction before they signed up to prescribe buprenorphine. It has proven valuable for some narcotic addicts, but for others, with addiction to nonopioid agents like alcohol, it has no effect.

The introduction of buprenorphine has moved the culture of medical addiction treatment away from the option of investing in the use of psychosocial options, such as Narcotics Anonymous or AA in particular. In fact, income is generated from writing buprenorphine prescriptions rather than spending time encouraging patients to go to NA or AA. Although pharmacology may have much to offer the treatment of addictive disorders, this shift in emphasis has meant that there is less attention given to nonpharmacologic recovery approaches, which themselves can be beneficial, alone or in combination with medications. This is unfortunate, particularly for young people for whom a drug-free Twelve-Step-based recovery from opioids at a relatively early age may be a better approach in the long run. One study showed excellent maintenance for adolescent opioid addicts on buprenorphine for a period of twelve weeks.[11] When I discussed the outcome of the study with its author, though, he was clear in acknowledging that after the drug trial period, virtually all the subjects in the study relapsed back to opioid addiction.

What, then, might be a reasonable perspective for the use of maintenance medications by doctors and concomitant use of Twelve Step recovery? AA has come around to the position that it is "wrong to deprive any alcoholic of any medication which can alleviate or control disabling physical and/or emotional problems." The NA position is that taking medication is to be determined by members in consultation with their sponsors and their respective NA groups.[12] In any given group, members may not fully accept someone on opioid maintenance, given that complete abstinence from maintenance drugs is generally their goal.

One needs to be sensitive to these issues and respectful of the concern that opioid maintenance, unlike medications such as antidepressants, may bring out the objection of members in some, even most, Twelve Step meetings. The door, however, does seem to be opening to consideration of maintenance drugs as acceptable in some Twelve Step groups. Overall, it seems most appropriate that this issue be left between member and sponsor, rather than in open discussion. Because many opioid-addicted people abuse alcohol and other drugs, a Twelve Step experience can certainly be valuable for them.

Change comes slowly in a fellowship like AA, where the use of "group conscience" for decision-making means that a minority, even a single individual, can successfully object to a new position for the group. In one respect this is useful, because it protects the integrity of a program whose absolute spiritual commitment can be made vulnerable by rapid modification. In other respects, it means that adaptation to new circumstances may come very slowly. Clearly there is a need for better collaboration between doctors and members of the Twelve Step community.

CHAPTER 10

The Rehabs

A A has indeed sustained its tradition of not being run by professionals, but its success has spawned residential programs that are now
operated by professionals and by business people. We can consider several
different recovery-oriented residential settings of this type. They typically house addicted people for a month, sometimes more. Each of these
has something to tell us about how the AA/NA model has influenced its
development. They also have some things to tell us about where Twelve-
Step-based recovery stands today. We can begin with one such program
that best illustrates a nonprofit institution dedicated to integrating AA
into the recovery process.

The rehabilitation programs, "rehabs," began with the Hazelden
Foundation, located in Center City, Minnesota. In 1948, with charitable
support, a recovering alcoholic established a treatment center for chronic
alcoholics on a 217-acre farm.[1] It was initially led by a recovering manager, and most of its early residents were chronic alcoholics from the
Minneapolis–St. Paul area. Its program included lectures and group meetings, with a strong focus on the Twelve Steps. With careful management
and access to professionals, Hazelden has grown into a multiunit facility
where residents can stay for three to four weeks, sometimes longer, taking
advantage of the variety of treatment modalities it offers. But again, its
operating philosophy was built around an emphasis on Twelve-Step-based
recovery.

Its format came to be known as "The Minnesota Model," and has been
applied in many settings across the United States and overseas. It was
initially the standard for residential facilities oriented toward alcoholism
recovery, and later, recovery from other drugs as well. In effect, it provided

a technology by which AA could be wedded to professional care, even if AA meetings were themselves independent of the professional managers. Physicians are employed to assure proper medical care, and this validates at least some insurance reimbursement for this treatment model. Importantly, physicians in the community more broadly have come to see rehabs like Hazelden as a resource for alcoholic and drug-addicted patients whom they are unable to manage on an outpatient basis.

The Minnesota Model, therefore, created a professional basis for the use of AA within a formally structured residential program. It also provided a model for cooperative work between alcoholism counselors, most of whom were in recovery, and professionals such as social workers, psychologists, and physicians. The Minnesota Model integrates a number of professional modalities into its program, which is infused with the AA philosophy of spiritually grounded abstinence. These include individual counseling, education about addiction, counseling groups for family members, and relapse prevention training. Twelve Step meetings are held both on and off the campus.

For a number of reasons, this model has been successful in spawning similar programs in the States and overseas, particularly in Great Britain and Scandinavia. "Twelfth Step work" means "to carry this message to other alcoholics." The Minnesota Model does this through an institution rather that through individuals, thereby allowing for proselytizing, which individual members do not do. It can, therefore, provide trainings for professionals, even in Minnesota, in the form of a degree-granting program. Hazelden itself supports a publishing arm that markets books addressing many different aspects of Twelve Step recovery, from the history of AA to personal tales of affected individuals.

This model also offered recovering people a way of transforming their personal support of other alcoholics to an institutional structure, and with charitable support as appropriate. For example, Richard Caron was a wealthy industrialist who had been treated at Hazelden. After returning home to Pennsylvania he would welcome alcoholics to sit around in his home and "chit chat" to fortify their early recovery. As more alcoholics would turn to him, he opened Chit Chat Farms in 1957 on a hotel property that he purchased. The Minnesota Model he had witnessed in his own recovery served to provide a system for the support he wanted to provide. From this start, there emerged the Caron Foundation, with programs located in sites across the Eastern United States.

The emergence and growth of this model can be considered from a sociologic perspective. Dissemination of the Hazelden technology was fueled by the creed of the AA, as personified in Bill W and the zeal of those who experienced the redemption he espoused. This evangelism has characterized movements from early Christian sects to contemporary social activist activities. Even the concept of socialism, dedicated to the idea of communal ownership of the means of production has had broad application by zealous leaders since early in the twentieth century. As sociologist Max Weber theorized,[2] such movements begin with charismatic zeal, usually under the leadership of a revered person. Later, they may spawn an organizational structure in which the original charismatic zeal is invested, such as the clergy of a church.

In order to survive, such a system needs to adapt to changing circumstances, and in the case of the Minnesota Model, this has taken the form of scientifically grounded advances in treatment. Counselors there now employ more recently developed therapeutic approaches such as cognitive behavioral therapy and dialectical behavior therapy. Medications for depression or even for psychotic symptoms are dispensed as needed. The introduction of these treatment advances not only serves patients well, but also assures that the underlying Twelve Step ideology will be acceptable in an evolving professional culture, thereby assuring broader societal support in the form of monetary expenditure.

An even further extension of this professionalization is the emergence of the Twelve Step rehabilitation facilities affiliated with academic medical centers. This integration is seen, for example, at the University of Florida in Gainesville, where resources include a medically grounded detoxification program, a residential rehab, and an academic teaching facility. Upon discharge, patients treated here can be referred to formally trained addiction psychiatrists or internists.

The Minnesota Model, therefore, also has been open to the use of medications for psychiatric disorders, particularly as the mentally ill increasingly have fallen prey to using alcohol and drugs to allay the distressing symptoms produced by their illnesses. Another opening for the use of medications has come about from Hazelden offering the opioid maintenance drug buprenorphine for heroin and narcotic pill addicts, along with recovery based on the Twelve Step model. This is particularly innovative relative to the AA philosophy of abstinence, because buprenorphine, although lifesaving for many addicted people, is itself a dependence-producing drug. It was a rather bold move when Dr. Marvin Seppala, the Hazelden medical director, decided to introduce this option when he saw how many of his Hazelden opioid-dependent patients were suffering overdoses after discharge from his facility.

The rehabs, however, are controversial. Studies showing that outpatient treatment and inpatient treatment in some settings may not differ in outcome raise questions about the considerable expense of residential rehab stays. In addition, the introduction of evidence-based treatments (those tested with randomization), such as cognitive behavioral therapy and motivational enhancement, have offered systematic alternatives to just staying put in a residential setting.

On the positive side, rehabs are a resource for addicted people who cannot limit their drinking and drug use while they are outpatients, even with a highly supportive clinic structure. In such cases, these inpatient programs may be needed to protect some alcoholics and addicts from severe medical consequences, serious accidents, or overdose. Professionals who have doubts about the effectiveness of the Minnesota Model point out that only a few positive studies on it have been carried out, such as one conducted at Hazelden.[3] In another study, patients randomly assigned to an outpatient Minnesota Model Program in comparison to public treatment were more likely to be abstinent over a twelve-month treatment period. The difference declined, however, after the one year of follow-up, suggesting the need for better ongoing support for Twelve Step alumni after the initial period of care.[4]

Another issue that has left rehabs open to questions is the emergence of the luxury-oriented programs that have sprung up to treat wealthy and celebrity types. There are no less than thirty-five for-profit, state-licensed rehabs in the city of Malibu (population: 12,645), California, many with scenic views overlooking the Pacific Ocean.[5] Some offer an array of untested treatment options, ranging from equine therapy (relating to horses in a therapeutic manner) to neurofeedback (employing unrelated neuroimaging information), to Qigong Chinese techniques. These rehabs are attractive to those who can afford them, but their cost can be more than twice that of long-established, nonprofit programs like Hazelden. Many offer creature comforts well worth the luxury hotel rates. Many let their residents go out into the community at will for whatever they may choose to do, or to partake of only those aspects of treatment that appeal to them. Some do make use of AA as a resource, but may not list this too prominently in their promotional materials for fear that an expectation of abstinence might scare some people off.

Given the diversity among rehab programs, the unproven nature of their outcomes, and for many, little if any relation to doctors practicing research-based techniques, what can we expect for the rehab universe in the future? No doubt many people in recovery owe their well-being to the rehabs, but whether rehabs represent the most efficient and effective approach for many who sign up is open to question. Many rehabs are a long way from employing a systematized and biomedically grounded approach to treatment, unlike what we see in long-established residential programs developed to treat the mentally ill.

One example of the uncertain economic circumstances that can beset the rehabs was evident in one of the most famous of them, the Betty Ford Center, in Rancho Mirage, California. Problems in filling its beds resulted less from questions of the value of residential treatment than from the availability of alternative luxurious options for people seeking out residential programs. When Elizabeth Taylor, one of Betty Ford's earliest celebrity residents, had been admitted, she had to sleep in the four-bedded room along with other residents, and help with cleanup responsibilities. These are "indignities" that patients no longer suffer when they decide to get help for their substance abuse, and they have the option of going elsewhere. Given its economic circumstances, the Betty Ford Center affiliated with the Hazelden Foundation to stabilize its economic situation. This combined nonprofit system now has a network of sixteen sites spread across the country, from California to New York to Florida.

It is interesting to consider how the rehabs might evolve into progressive networks of treatment programs, with components tailored to various types of addictive disorders and severities. The Sheppard and Enoch Pratt Health System was founded in 1853 in Baltimore, Maryland as a progressive and comfortable retreat for mentally ill people whose affluent families and doctors were at a loss as to how to manage them. Over the years, the concept of support and comfort for those referred has not been forsaken, and it is now infused into a network of thirty-eight psychiatrically sophisticated treatment centers in the greater Baltimore area. The system, headed by a past president of the American Psychiatric Association, has been ranked among the top psychiatric facilities nationally.[6] Perhaps such an evolution will take place in the addiction rehab field.

Most rehabs, though, if reporting honestly, indicate that many who complete their programs relapse soon after discharge, often within a month. There are good reasons for this, principal among them that we do not have definitive treatments for addiction. Often, more extensive residential experience is needed to stabilize some addicted people. Multiple admissions may be needed.

Additionally, treatment follow-up after discharge is often unreliable. The programs are usually not located in the city where the admitted person lives, and competent aftercare, ideally in the hands of an expert professional, may not be readily available when they return home. Even if it is available, the hand-to-hand transfer from the residential facility to post-discharge treatment is often not reliably arranged, and people sometimes do not even call the professional with whom they were supposed to follow up; many leave glad to think they have done enough already.

Furthermore, although most rehabs provide a reasonable introduction to the Twelve Step approach, AA and NA are not "treatments." Treatment is provided by professionals, and for addicted people not fully stabilized, a competently framed, professionally managed program is essential. Intensive outpatient programs that include medications as appropriate can help to fill this need.

A less intensive Twelve-Step-oriented residential stay also can provide needed support, by continuing the therapeutic culture of the rehab experience. An example of this is the Serenity program, which operates residences in Manhattan. The program is not for "treatment," which is left in the hands of a referring professional. Residents there sleep in the facility, meals are served them, and they are expected to attend Twelve Step meetings in the community. With consultation from a case manager, they are expected to arrange appropriate activities during the day, be it work or volunteering. Given the Manhattan location, and the extent of the program, however, a one-month stay can cost $10,000.

Then there is the issue that rehabs themselves are quite expensive. Unlike government or Veterans Administration supported facilities, they typically range from $25,000 a month to as much as twice that when more amenities are offered. They employ professional staff with a master's degree or higher. Many meet specific requirements of certifying bodies, such as the Joint Commission that accredits healthcare organizations like hospitals. Their services are generally not covered by insurers, and for most people this comes to more than they can afford.

Are there less costly options? Can the volunteerism embodied in AA be extended so that Twelve Step members can provide a protective environment without a professionally driven format? In discussing Step Twelve, we considered the potential of lay people serving in therapist-like roles for people who have had the same illness as their own, addiction in this case. There is a model that merits consideration here, because it represents such an option. The spontaneity and enthusiasm of its founder was telling:

The way we started we were at the NA campout one week, sitting around the campfire. We said we need to start something. On that Monday, I went to see a lawyer, and called my wife and told her what I was doing. She was a bit surprised, but I just asked her what she wanted to name it. Came up with the name McShin. She's McDaid and I'm Shinholser, and I filled out the 501(c3) and put it in the mail the same day. I went over to a treatment center I knew in the city, and asked if I could rent a space. So I rented a 56-square-foot office and we quickly outgrew it. Now we're in a 15,000-square-foot facility. What happened when word got out that I was helping people full-time, was that we just got inundated with people.

Who was providing the support services, and supervision?

We were just recovering people trying to help people recover. Strictly all volunteers, peer-to-peer, you join and you teach one. Kinda like the principles of the Twelve Step program. Except instead of doing it one hour per night, we did it basically sixteen hours a day.

McShin had moved to larger space in the wing of a local church and began locating people in houses they rented nearby. This was a "peer-to-peer" operation, which came to rely primarily on the voluntary commitment of stabilized addicted people to supervise residents in each of four houses where supervisors are given free room and board. Because the houses are not locked facilities, urine toxicologies are conducted to monitor residents for drugs of abuse. Given their experiences, McShin developed a manual for "recovery coaches," one that has been disseminated widely on the Internet.

Most of the operation's expenses are covered by a modest fee, currently $4,800 for a first month. Residents can then stay on for $125 a week. A more extensive first-month program, with visits from a physician, himself in recovery, and a weekly session with a certified addiction counselor, costs $8,700, still no more than a third of the cost for the least expensive formally certified rehabs. The facility president, whose expertise is drawn solely from his own recovery, oversees it with great dedication, and solicits outside contributions, which amount to a third of the program's operating budget. This program and several others like it have established a Council on Accreditation of Peer Recovery Support Services.

Is this a model that can be replicated more widely? Are such programs, relying heavily on the dedication and good sense of their founders, a viable option to shelter people in a system that does not have professional management? This might be answered affirmatively in settings where dedicated leadership and low-cost physical facilities are available, and where alternatives are not available.

However ubiquitous Twelve Step groups are, the availability of residential treatment is clearly limited relative to the actual need. This is particularly the case for disadvantaged people with combined mental illness and addiction. One cost-effective approach to this problem that we developed for our Bellevue patients in New York was a Twelve-Step-oriented program in the adjacent shelter for the homeless. This example illustrates again how less costly programs can be initiated, and how they can be considered when an appropriate opportunity arises. The program was embedded in one wing of a nearby homeless shelter, drawing on support for room and board available there, and appending onto it the staff of a low-intensity outpatient program, one that took advantage of Twelve Step meetings. It also embodied a peer-led therapeutic community program that we had initiated with George DeLeon, an expert in therapeutic communities. We found the staff well able to bridge the formats of mental illness treatment and the peer-led therapeutic model for addiction.[7] Although many of these chronically homeless patients had records of arrest, their clinical outcome, again with dedicated staff support, was no different from that of those without such records.[8]

Institutional restraints are hard to overcome. Our program in the homeless shelter, for example, was always vulnerable to the overall shelter administration, which bore no sympathy toward our deviation from their usual format. When we tried to establish a casual walk-in format for the program's graduates in the hospital itself, we found that no staff member could participate unless we instituted an elaborate system of medical charting and payments that paralleled those of the medical clinics, and this option was not workable. Nonetheless, the impulse toward Twelve-Step-based volunteerism carries with it a zeal that will always gravitate toward opportunities to "carry the message."

Most rehabs have a long way to go in terms of effective programming. By employing the Twelve Step format that is at the core of most of them, they have been beneficial for many whose lives have been saved. But there is not yet any standardized research-based approach developed for rehab treatment, and many of the facilities' leaders have little relationship with the established medical organizations that focus on careful and thoughtful research-based management for addicted people. On the other hand, for many addicted people these residential programs have provided the material benefit of recovery, and given the fact that addiction treatment is an evolving field, the future of this approach may turn out to be quite positive.

CHAPTER 11

How it Changes the Brain

Not long after my residency in psychiatry, while I was starting out in the addiction field, I went to speak about alcoholism and drug problems with the chairman of the pathology department at my medical school. He was a wise and venerated man. At one point, while we were discussing AA, he asked me, "What is the mechanism?" He did not seem to be interested in my ideas about the psychology of what motivates people, which I tried to explain to him at the time. Later that day, I realized that for him, mechanisms were spelled out in physiologic and biochemical measures. But even in that day, his way of looking at things biologically was not removed from the domain of psychiatry. It was embedded in the thinking of Freud, the great student of human motivation, who was known for having said, "Anatomy is destiny." After all, Freud did start his career as a neuropathologist.

When doctors talk about biology in relation to treating addiction, they are most often referring to the bodily damage it does: Alcohol numbs the brain and causes illness through its toxic effect on organ systems, like the liver and heart. For drugs, we hear about heart arrhythmias from cocaine, or overdoses from heroin. We need treatments for these physical maladies (ideally in pill form), but for the time being, we are going to set those concerns aside, and consider instead some very different aspects of addiction. We will look at how AA relates to what we know about the biology of social interaction and its role in brain function.

Nowadays, hope exists that medical treatments will ultimately solve the problem of addiction, and maybe they will. In the case of alcoholism, there are some medications that impact body chemistry and decrease the likelihood of a return to heavy drinking, such as naltrexone, topiramate, and acamprosate, but these have been studied under controlled circumstances, that is to say, under protocols where participants are extensively evaluated and their subsequent drinking (or not drinking) followed up by teams of research staff. These drugs appear to alter drinking patterns somewhat more than do the placebo pills against which they are usually pitted. This seems promising, but in "real life," where a doctor does the prescribing, sends the patient home, or perhaps refers them to a counselor, people tend to stop taking the pills after a while. If we had the opportunity to follow each alcoholic over the long haul, we might see more of the benefit observed in these studies. But adherence to medications is found to be far from reliable for most illnesses, and for alcoholics, whose denial and likelihood of relapse is considerable, the long-term benefit of these drugs is still open to question. In fact, we have no long-term studies on the role of these medications for treating alcoholism. We do not know how many—if any—alcoholics keep taking them for, let's say, more than a year. Nor do we know whether taking these medications for a while, say a few months, outside of a highly structured protocol, impacts on whether alcoholics taking them would be better off a year or two later. Nonetheless, most of the members of the clinical research community strongly promote their use, and believe that long-term benefit would accrue.

Another biologic domain for research on addiction is the idea that focusing on the genetics of the illness will yield clues as to how a vulnerability to it is associated with particular gene loci. Studies on kids adopted from birth are revealing in this regard. The progeny of alcoholics, whether raised by the alcoholic natural parents or by non-alcoholic adoptive parents, have been found to have a much greater likelihood of becoming alcoholic than children born to non-alcoholics. The natural parents' genetic makeup is very influential. The vulnerability to alcoholism breeds true, and we are finding similar results for drug problems. Nonetheless, our research on the biology of this genetic vulnerability has been surprisingly unrevealing. Many millions of dollars were invested in the federal government's Collaborative Studies on the Genetics of Alcoholism project that was begun in the 1990s. Blood samples were drawn on thousands of people, but they have not yielded a genetic constellation that accounts for a sizable portion of the risk for developing the disease. Research continues on this with considerable support by the review committees at the National Institute of Alcohol Abuse and Alcoholism. We will see where it goes in studying a disease that is more complicated than we would like to believe.

Do we have evidence of long-term benefit from all these biomedically oriented investments? There are many people on opioid maintenance who have been freed from their use of heroin or their illegal use of pain pills, but other than that, the picture remains unclear. Let's just say that there has never been an attempt to tabulate how many addicted people are better off in the long run based on their use of numerous other medications.

How much research investment has the federal government put into the way AA works? Or into how its use could be promoted? Hardly a small fraction of what's gone into all the aforementioned biomedically oriented efforts. And is there any degree of zeal in the research community for promoting studies on AA? One would be hard-pressed to find many interested in such research among over a thousand attendees at the annual meetings of the Research Society on Alcoholism, most of whom are there on grant support from the federal government.

Why is this? Why do all of these researchers cohere around the biological models of pharmacology and genetic markers? Some insight into this can be gained in considering a concept developed by Thomas Kuhn, a historian of science. While teaching at the University of California, Berkeley in 1962, he wrote a book, *The Structure of Scientific Revolutions,*[1] in which he pointed out that at any given time, scientists in a particular area of research operate as a community adhering to a particular paradigm—a model for understanding—in their endeavors. Research within that paradigm yields findings that help illuminate the area under study. At some point, though, the yield of research employing that paradigm begins to run out; it is no longer fruitful. Soon a new paradigm for research may emerge, one that generates new findings. Eventually, a revolution of sorts takes place, after which research can be based on the new paradigm. Important to this model of scientific research is the following: The old paradigm need not be wrong; it may just be less fertile for new findings.

I would suggest, with regard to research on addiction recovery, that the community of scientists who cohere to the pharmacologic–genetic model are neither understanding of nor open to one built around the biology of social influence. Neither model is exclusively "right," but each reflects a valid perspective for scientific investigation. One community of researchers involved with the former—the pharmacogenetic model—are just predominating these days.

So here is what you, the reader, can consider in approaching this chapter. The pharmacologic–genetic paradigm for "getting better" from addiction has its own inherent merit, but there is another paradigm, a sociobiologic one, which needs to be considered in order to understand how AA works. Why is this? Because AA is a socially structured group built on feelings of affiliation and shared beliefs. There are ways of conducting or piecing together existing research within this latter paradigm that are more suited to understanding why folks in long-term abstinence, particularly those in AA, may become stable and no longer crave alcohol or drugs.

In order to pursue this line of research, we will consider how people's behavior can reflect reactions to their social environment that are rooted in their biology, and begin to look at how this plays out in brain function. I will try to explain all this in a way that relates participation in a group to the way a person's mind is influenced, all based on the biology of social behavior. We will consider two related aspects of this paradigm: sociobiology and neuroscience. Let me give you a taste of some issues that each discipline addresses.

Sociobiology is a discipline that was brought to wide attention by the entomologist Edward Wilson.[2] He knew full well that Darwin had revolutionized our understanding of how different species' physical structure and their respective organs evolved—from creatures who live in water to those who live on land, from fins for swimming to feet for walking. What Wilson synthesized from a large body of research was how behaviors, and not just body parts, evolve, and what the biologic basis of that behavioral evolution is. He explained that these behavioral changes evolve for the same reason that body parts do, to promote survival of the species. Take the progression from fins to feet. What is adaptive to survival of the species is that which assures that one's genes will be passed from one generation to the next. And presumably, this progression is rooted in biology, however complex it may be.

Primates as different as monkeys and humans have descended from common ancestors; members of both species tend to live together in groups, and they all innately respond to their young offspring by taking care of them after birth. These traits assure that one individual's genes will successfully pass on to the next generation. In relation to AA, we will try to understand how particular behaviors, such as people bonding together in a tightly knit group and acquiring shared beliefs, are adaptive, and how these behaviors were sustained as part of humans'—homo sapiens'—evolutionary adaptation.

We are interested here in those aspects of neural function that make for the social bonding and shared beliefs that characterize AA membership. In this respect we will have to look at the way brain and mind are bound together. Rene Descartes,[3] the seventeenth-century philosopher, struggled with this dualism: Are the mind and body separate entities that are independent of each other, or do they constitute one unified whole? Neuroscience is the research-based study of how the nervous system works. It will help us answer this question as best one can nowadays. Here are some examples of this discipline.

Cognitive neuroscience focuses on an aspect, organizing what people perceive, see, and hear, and then relates this to how they understand and think. On the level of one neuron, it helps us to understand a surprising finding like this: Brain surgeons operating on people with intractable epilepsy had to stimulate different areas of the cerebral cortex in order to locate a site that triggered a particular patient's seizures. Working with colleagues, Itzhak Fried[4] found that he could stimulate just one particular neuron that responded to only one kind of stimulus. In this case, it was pictures of the actress Jennifer Aniston. (A different neuron would only respond to pictures of Julia Roberts.) How does the mind remember Jennifer Aniston's image, in whatever pose she was presented? How does the concept of this woman get framed into a neural network that was tied to that one neuron? What kind of functional connections from that neuron underlie this? Is there a Bill W neuron for AA members? Cognitive neuroscience deals with how certain images and memories are established in the brain; how we understand sensations and attribute meaning to them.

On the other hand, *social* neuroscientists seek to find out how different brain centers are associated with certain social behaviors. We will be looking at findings related to AA in more detail, but here is an example that bears on behaviors that are reflected in what people do in AA: Infant monkeys will copy the actions of a person who is facing them. If a person sticks her tongue out in front of an infant monkey, that little creature may then stick out its own tongue. Humans, even in early infancy, will show this reaction as well. In human grown-ups, this can relate to sensing what another person feels, as opposed to merely perceiving their actions. This, in turn, relates to the complex capacity of experiencing empathy. This brain-based empathy can be considered an important aspect of the closeness and acceptance seen among AA members. Social behaviors can be traced to specific brain sites that are activated by mirroring or by empathy. Social behaviors like the fidelity and mutuality among AA members, we will find, can be understood to emerge from such brain sites.

SOCIOBIOLOGY

In *The Descent of Man*,[5] Charles Darwin expressed interest in developing an approach to psychology that would explain how and why similar social traits are found in very different species. He wrote, "with what care male birds display their various charms. . . . we ought not to accuse birds of conscious vanities; yet when we see a peacock strutting about, with expanded and quivering tail feathers, he seems the very emblem of pride and vanity."[6]

It was decades later that the study of animal behavior was being developed as an empirical science by Konrad Lorenz.[7] He considered innate social behaviors that could be found in very different species. Terms like "falling in love, marrying, or being jealous" could apply to pairs of geese that stay together the way human couples do.

Why do behaviors like these emerge over the course of evolution in different species? Apparently both geese and their human counterparts are genetically built to act in ways that assure the survival of their respective species. Among humans we see behaviors that appear across all cultures, like many maternal, sexual, and aggressive traits. They are so universal that we can assume that they somehow draw on inborn, instinctual, biologic roots. If this is so, then they must be adaptive in terms of promoting survival and, therefore, be carried from one generation to the next. In the case of understanding how AA "works," we will see how this relates to traits associated with the way people support each other in groups.

In a previous chapter we discussed how people become engaged in AA, and how groups of people can draw their members into observing the rituals they espouse. This can take place in charismatic, cult-like groups. In a less all-encompassing way, we looked at the psychology of spiritually oriented movements, of which AA is an example. In charismatic, cult-like groups, people behave with a certain rigidity. In the Unification Church, "Moonies" pretty much blindly followed the expectations of their charismatic leader, Rev. Moon. Members of the Hindu-derived cult, the Divine Light Mission, also would adhere to what their group's leader expected of them.

In studying these groups, we found that members' emotional well-being was dependent on the degree to which they felt socially attached to other members and accepted the groups' beliefs. If asked to, members would sacrifice for the group and for their fellow members. In addition, the malaise they felt before joining would be relieved relative to their commitment and participation in the group.[3]

The pattern of one's equanimity being related to ties to one's social group can be seen as related to the human trait of altruism. Altruism is an innate trait in humans (and some other species) that suggests a seeming paradox: Altruistic behavior would seem to compromise a person, even limiting his capacity to reproduce, and thereby limit how his genes would be passed on to ensuing generations. Ethologists were puzzled as to how a trait that could limit an individual's own ability to pass its genes on could persist over the course of evolution.

The altruist who tries to save a drowning swimmer, and might thereby lose his life in the process, has one thing in common with the person who becomes engaged in the charismatic group. From an evolutionary standpoint, both sacrifice their individual interests and survival potential for the benefit of others; they may diminish their chance to reproduce by virtue of carrying that trait. This raises the question of how such traits persist over the course of evolution, in spite of the fact that carriers may be less likely to survive and transmit the genes to the next generation.

Consider the following. A trait observed in a given individual may serve to improve the reproductive advantage of other related individuals who may carry genes for that same trait. This would apply to a person's sibling with half the likelihood of carrying the same genes for that behavior—or to an uncle with one quarter of that chance. That way, an altruist who helps a sibling or uncle survive is promoting the transmission of the altruist gene through this relative. This takes place even if the altruist himself does not produce progeny because of sacrificing his chance for survival. This principle of population genetics is called inclusive fitness (as opposed to individual fitness).

The concept of inclusive fitness goes to the heart of sociobiology. As proposed by William D. Hamilton,[9] this form of genetic fitness reflects not only the fitness of a given individual carrying a genetic trait, but also the fitness of all that individual's relatives who might carry the genes for that trait, since their survival also ensures the trait's transmission. Inclusive fitness can therefore allow a social trait to persist in a species, even if it does not persist in that individual carrier.

We can also consider the concept of reciprocal altruism here. Robert Trivers[10] pointed out that an altruistic trait need not only be based on the advantage it gives the actual relatives who are assisted. It can reflect the reciprocal benefits in a family or a larger population of remotely related individuals who act toward each other in an altruistic way. That way they assure some measure of reciprocity when that person may later be in need. As you can see, all this helps to explain the survival of traits that do not necessarily endow a given individual with greater genetic fitness.

And here is how it can operate in practice: When people become involved in a charismatic group, the closer they feel tied into the group, the less distress they feel. Conversely, if they consider removing themselves from the group a bit, they are prodded to not do so by an increase in the amount of distress they are likely to feel. This way, zealous group members feel unhappy when removed from their group. Committed members of a group like Alcoholics Anonymous, for example, often report feeling uneasy or out of sorts when they miss a number of meetings.

Group members are, therefore, poised between a reward for closeness and a negative pressure for alienation. Each minor episode of reward or punishment, upon moving closer to the group or moving further away, functions as a learning experience. In terms of behavioral psychology, this is called operant reinforcement. It habituates (conditions) involvement. The process is similar to a conditioning experiment in which an animal is rewarded each time it carries out a particular behavior. A mouse can be rewarded with cheese every time it taps a lever. Eventually, it will keep tapping the lever even if the bits of cheese are few and far between.

A charismatic group member is like a human subject in an operant conditioning study, where she or he is being reinforced to stay involved as a member. This can occur even without the person being aware of it. Similarly, the malaise associated with feelings of alienation tends to make members avoid distancing themselves from the group. A new group member, undergoing this process, will continue in a pattern of maintaining closeness even if rewards are provided only intermittently. This effect thereby serves as reinforcement for continued group involvement. My point is that this is biologically grounded.

Close ties among members of a social group also are seen in nonhuman primates. Such ties are common in the community organization of chimpanzees in the wild, who migrate, collaborate, and stay close to one another in bands.[11] In research studies, a young monkey can be removed from the cage where it has lived with other young monkeys, with whom it had been raised, and left alone in another cage. Eventually it exhibits a decrease in activity, a doleful expression, and a crouched posture. Severing the bonds that this monkey had to the peers in its social network produces behaviors similar to those seen with depression in humans. But when the isolated monkey is introduced into a new group of young monkeys, this "depression" is relieved. Interestingly, a biologic intervention produces the same effect of relief from depression. Giving the isolated monkey an antidepressant medication, even without returning it to a peer group, relieves those signs of depression.[12] Here we see a bridging of the social and biologic models.

BIOLOGY AND THE BRAIN

Let's now consider some of the ways that this sociobiologic model might open up consideration of brain science. Australopithecus hominids, direct ancestors of Homo sapiens, inhabited forested areas of East Africa from about five million to one million years ago. Over many generations they developed stable patterns of group social organization in order to assume adequate nutrition by hunting large game.[13] As hominids evolved, their cranial capacities doubled between the time of the australopithecine era and the appearance about a million years ago of Homo erectus, a more recent human precursor.[14] Such massive increases, in cortical matter primarily, have underlain significant changes in the behavioral repertoires of our hominid ancestors.

So what may go on in the brain relative to AA? We can first consider why contemporary humans developed an enlarged brain over evolutionary time. For one thing, the brain is an active organ. Although it makes up only 2% of body weight it consumes ten times that percentage of the body's total energy intake. Not all parts of the brain grew larger at an equal rate. Ethologists have found that the more complex the social order in a primate species, the larger the neocortex, the component of the brain associated with understanding and reasoning. And studies have shown that much of this enhanced growth in humans took place in regions of the brain related to social and interpersonal skills. This has been termed the social brain hypothesis.[15]

There is a famous case of an injury that illustrates the location of these social functions in the frontal lobes of the neocortex. Phineas Gage was a railroad worker who experienced a horrible accident: An explosion shot a metal rod through his head and into his neocortex. It did not kill him or result in a loss of his IQ, perception, or memory skills, but although he had been a polite and socially appropriate person before the accident, his behavior changed dramatically afterward. He became uncaring, profane, and socially inappropriate.[16] In a way, the loss that he experienced relates to experiencing oneself and others as real sentient entities, and acting appropriately.

What innate interpersonal skills did humans acquire that lower primates did not? One interesting experiment[17] was undertaken to test this. Chimpanzees and orangutans were compared to two-and-a-half-year-old children in a laboratory setting using a primate test battery. The chimpanzees, orangutans, and human children all performed the same on tests of intelligence related to physical objects, such as being able to distinguish two from three toys presented them, but the human children had advanced more in skills associated with sociality. They outperformed the chimpanzees and orangutans in social learning, like understanding gestures made by the experimenters. It seems that social interaction is where the biggest differences began to emerge early on in evolution, as man became smarter and his brain size increased.

So let's look at which brain functions operate in relation to the complex social interactions that take place in AA. In trying to shed light on a spiritual fellowship like AA, why would we tie together biologic models as remote from each other as animal behavior and the way neurons interact? What I hope will become clear is that there is a scientific paradigm that can be seen to emerge from this body of research that answers the question posed by the pathology chairman I spoke with at the beginning of this chapter, when he asked, "What is the mechanism behind AA?" It may be that by extending findings from social and cognitive neuroscience to an evolutionary model, we can better understand some of the ways to cope with addictive illnesses, including the use of AA.

Joining a close-knit group can be adaptive from an evolutionary standpoint. One can certainly say that the kind of social behavior associated with Twelve Step groups is adaptive, in that members who support one another in staying sober live a healthier life, and live longer. We found that one aspect of this adaptation is the way the long-term members we surveyed experienced little or no craving for alcohol or drugs. We got the same story from similar members in our focus groups who volunteered to discuss their experiences.

I began to wonder just what was going on psychologically and physiologically with these folks that their cravings seem to have been quieted, given that the usual models from classical psychology, such as conditioning and cognitive behavior therapy, did not seem to fully capture this. It was clear that major changes in these members' motivation for sobriety and the way they lived their lives had taken place. The question was: How did this translate into being liberated from the compelling alcohol craving that they had struggled with before joining the fellowship?

One way to approach this was to turn to the latest findings on brain research that might be associated with this, because this research was apparently at the frontier of contemporary psychology. These breakthroughs in technique came from looking at what the brain is doing in people while they are actually awake, thinking, and feeling. The technology for detecting this had resulted from the invention of magnetic resonance imaging (MRI) for which the Nobel Prize was awarded in 2003. It works by creating a very strong magnetic field surrounding the person being studied. This makes the protons in the hydrogen atoms in tissue that contains water generate a signal that can then be processed to show which areas differ in their water density. It ends up looking something like an X-ray. Because bones have much less water in them than soft tissue, they show up differently on the scan. This is particularly valuable in studying the brain itself because its various components differ from each other in water density.

By using this approach researchers can now see which brain areas are activated at a given time. This works because when a brain area is activated, it uses more oxygen, and the oxygen concentration in that area can now be measured. We will be reviewing a number of studies that employ this functional Magnetic Resonance Imaging (fMRI) technique to show where different activities take place in respective areas of the brain.

There are some points we should consider before we begin. The first is that in describing these studies, I will not specify the names of the specific components that were studied (like the dorsolateral prefrontal cortex), because these complicated designations are beyond the scope of this book. If you are interested in the particulars, you can refer to a technical article that I wrote about this.[18]

Another point is one of methodology. The fMRI research that I am citing was done in the laboratory, and a good deal of inference is needed to extend the findings to real-life situations. This limitation is due to the fact that one cannot carry a several-ton fMRI lab into a bar or an AA meeting. We will always be limited by the need to extrapolate from the lab to "real life."

Finally, most of the brain research on craving has been done on recently detoxified addicted people because, frankly, it is easier to get access to them than to long-term members, as alcohol and drug addicted people are most available when they are in treatment programs. This captures the acute changes that take place around the time of alcohol or drug use, but we are interested here in people who have been sober for a long time to see how their thinking has changed.

Here is a very condensed view of what happens in the *newly* admitted patients, rather than long-term members. It is widely touted as key to the addiction process. Drug ingestion itself increases release of dopamine, a neurotransmitter, but prolonged use alters certain dopamine receptors in certain areas at the base of the brain that moderate basic drives, like hunger and sex. This, in turn, leads to a compromise in the regulation of the brain circuitry that would otherwise moderate a response to the drug. And this then leaves heavy drug or alcohol users feeling a craving when they are exposed to a drug trigger. It has been found that this abnormality declines if one stays off drugs for a while, perhaps a few months.[19]

But we know that craving and relapse, prominent in people even after leaving treatment, is decreased in the long-term AA members. In order to consider why this might be, we can turn to recent fMRI research. This technology has been adopted widely because it can reveal brain activity sites without a researcher having to stick needles into people to inject contrast materials, or exposing them to potentially noxious X-rays. It has allowed for the expansion of two areas of research we are considering here, social neuroscience and cognitive neuroscience. Social neuroscience was developed by investigators[20] who initially began looking at hormonal changes associated with various aspects of communication and social influence, and then picked up on fMRI techniques as they became available to expand on this work. Cognitive neuroscience, as we said, deals with thinking, memory, and integrating complex concepts.

We can begin this exploration by looking at mirroring, a basic trait associated with social interaction that is observed in many primates, from monkeys to Homo sapiens. Earlier in this chapter, I mentioned mirror neurons, a phenomenon first noted in the early 1990s by Italian investigators[21] who were studying brain sites activated when monkeys reached for a piece of food. To their surprise, a brain site that related to the monkey itself picking up the food was detected when a monkey saw a person nearby pick up a piece of food. This has been termed mirroring.

In people, this has been elaborated as evolving into complex aspects of social interaction. It relates to processes that underlie how people perceive one another and sense other people's feelings and motivations. This intuitive process is called mentalizing, a concept that was developed early on in the psychoanalytic literature.[22] Clinicians posited that this process underlies how people, say a patient and a therapist, can experience feelings and thoughts together when in a session. Even before there was actual experimental evidence to back it up, mentalizing was thought to serve as a basis for the empathic exchanges that can take place in therapy sessions or among people in general.

With the use of fMRI, mentalizing has been shown to take place in particular brain sites. Consider a study in which subjects were asked about their own attitudes and those of another person: "How likely are you to think that keeping a diary is important?" versus "How likely is the Queen to think a diary is important?"[23] (Not surprisingly, this was done in Great Britain.) Then they also were asked, "How likely are you to sneeze when a cat is nearby?" and then "How likely is the Queen to sneeze when a cat is nearby?" The investigators were able to localize the subjects' brain activity in sites related to understanding another person's motivation as compared to their own. The investigators also could distinguish between areas related to sensing another person's spontaneous movement (the Queen sneezes) as opposed to her motivations (about a diary). Mentalizing was associated with the thinking about the another person's feelings and motivations, something like what goes on in the therapy session or among close-knit AA members, like a sponsor and sponsee.

Studies like this also distinguish the greater concern felt for those whom one considers close to oneself, as opposed to others who are not in one's in-group. This was done by having people, while in the scanner, respond to images related to relieving pain in players of their favorite soccer team compared with relieving pain in members of the opposing team,[24] and these differences could be localized as well. What we see here is a parallel to the neural basis for the concern felt by AA members for one another and doing "Twelve Step work," that is, acting on concern for people they feel close to, such as other alcoholics, compared to concern for non-alcoholics. The alcoholics are, as it were, on their team.

All this can be related to a quandary we considered that the philosopher Descartes first introduced some five hundred years ago: Where do mind and body (or mind and brain) intersect?[25] Neuroscientists are trying to answer this age-old question with studies like the ones we just considered. They talk about Theory of Mind, the ability to attribute mental states—beliefs, feelings, thoughts—to oneself and also to others; that way, you distinguish between the "you" and another person. This relates to reflecting on one's own motives and being able to imagine motives and feelings in others, like the Queen or the soccer players in those studies.[26] It also suggests a neural basis for empathy within the sphere of AA members.

To recap: We are trying to understand AA in biological terms. Empathic communication between members, sponsor and sponsee in particular, are a key element of AA function. In line with this, it has been pointed out that empathic exchanges have been important elements in the evolutionary adaptation of the human species. The processes of mentalizing, experience sharing, and empathic concern apparently became functionally integrated in the brain over evolutionary time.[27] These skills were adaptive because they allow for carrying out complex social tasks and interpersonal activities.

The ability to remember one's past experiences also influences the capacity for social interaction. This was evident in the brain-damaged person, Phineas Gage,[28] who experienced a loss of his own personal memories, which compromised his ability to behave appropriately with family and friends. His interactions with them became awkward, unpredictable, and often bizarre. He could not make judgments about what to say or how to act socially without being able to retrieve his own personal memories. We need to remember who we are in order to interact appropriately with others.

This brings us to the complex role of memory in the arena we are exploring. In the case of this brain-damaged person, the two separate sites for mentalizing and later remembering should have been associated with each other through a neural network, but the connections were severed. For other people, this is not a problem. AA members are exposed to plenty of situations where the ideas and expectations of AA are expressed, in meetings and in talking with other members. So we can look at how the social environment influences the way the brain remembers experiences like these and translates them into changing people's outlook on themselves or on their understanding about how to act like a sober alcoholic.

Imaging in the scanner can distinguish the remembering that one consciously undertakes—"Let me see, what did happen yesterday?"—from skills and activities that are remembered without even thinking, like how to ride a bicycle or how to interact with people. These two different kinds of skills are each summoned up from different brain networks. The latter type of unconsciously available memories, those we are considering here, can be laid down without one's knowing it, given the right environment (in our case, the AA social setting), and they can then influence future behavior. Processes like these have been spelled out by mapping these functions in their respective brain regions.

Memories also can be manipulated by environmental cues. Studies have been carried out associating pictures of faces of different people with pictures of particular places, like a house or a forest. When the place-related cues are switched around, the subjects' responses can change to alter how the faces are perceived. This happens without the experimental subject being aware that this is happening: The setting determines what memories the brain brings up.[29] Other sites can then act on memories and translate them into motivation and decision-making.[30] All this can take place outside a person's awareness. Things can be perceived differently when a person is engaged in a particular environment in real life and exposed to social influence.

This can come into play in a situation like brainwashing, a process that was studied in depth with regard to American GIs taken prisoner by the North Korean Communist regime during the Korean War. Some of them were transformed into spokesmen for their captors. Robert Lifton[31] described how control over the context of communication, the social environment these GIs were exposed to, could contribute to transforming them into true believers. In our own studies on the Unification Church, we found that an induction group's structure and influence determined the beliefs and attitudes that could be expressed there. This then led to some of the attendees becoming members of a sect that made exceptional demands on how they would run their lives.

In a more benign way, we see here how certain brain sites can be effectively engaged and orchestrated in the context of committed belief in the AA setting. People do give up (harmful) attitudes and behaviors to which they had been committed. And, as illustrated experimentally in the fMRI laboratory studies, this can be localized in specific sites, while it is taking place outside the awareness of the person exposed to social cues.

In the early twentieth century, the psychologist Jean Piaget[32] framed a model for how young children develop complex concepts, as when an infant is exposed to many different sensory inputs. In the case of its mother, for example, these inputs are visual, tactile, and nurturing. All these must be integrated into an overall conception in order for the infant to deal with and react to its "mother" as a coherent person. Such perceptions and feelings when integrated together are termed schemas.

Mental schemas allow us to understand the world around us in an integrated way. They are now coming to be explained in terms of the complex neural networks that embody them. This takes place once new information is acquired; it can be manipulated, recombined, and reordered in the development of a complex schema. Research on this process shows which brain sites are engaged in producing such self-contained memory structures, or schemas. The schemas can be associated with particular values (sobriety is good), and they then can frame the way new memories are acquired and expressed.[34] So when value judgments are exercised, as in what is right or wrong to do, this brain activity can be detected with scanning.[35]

It is important to note that these memory structures can come about outside the awareness of an individual, and that they also can embody emotional content.[36] In addition, they can be associated with a disposition that relates to decreased alcohol craving. This stands in contrast to the process of conscious suppression of craving, which also has been tracked by scanning.[37] Significantly for the long-term AA member, new schemas could embody a different view of oneself vis-à-vis drinking.

The concept of a self-schema[38] is important here, because a person carries a conception of herself, who she is, how she got there, and how she knows herself to act.[39] In the case of alcoholics, these self-schemas embody an identity as someone who needs to drink, as someone who will respond to triggers by seeking out alcohol. By intertwining one's life experience with the AA program, one's self-schema can be changed to a person who eschews alcohol. I wanted to look at how this comes about.

After trying to badger recalcitrant alcoholics to consider abstinence, Bill W concluded that the best way to approach them was to tell them his own story. The Big Book describes how he engaged potential AA members by offering a series of first-person accounts, the stories of people who found their way to recovery in AA. In a similar way, sponsors tell sponsees their own stories in the course of encouraging them to work the Steps. In fact, the most common format for AA meetings is built around self-disclosure stories of speakers as they "qualify," that is, go up to speak to those assembled. These stories reinforce participants' acquisition of a shared identity as recovering alcoholics.[40] This leads to the reshaping of a member's self-schema through repeated exposure in the social context to a different view of oneself. One's self-schema is gradually transformed in the context of social communication and influence. In fact, self-disclosure has been found to be strongly associated with reward activation in certain brain regions, thereby reinforcing the inclination of people toward self-revelation.[41]

The Twelve-Step approach to recovery is distinguished from professionally grounded treatments like cognitive behavioral therapy by one of its most prominent features: It conveys a system of values that extends beyond just being abstinent. One sees this when members are expected to consider their own role in problems they previously had blamed on other people (Step Four) and later, when they are expected to make amends to the people they had harmed (Step Nine). This has its counterpart in lab studies in which people are asked to make decisions that draw on their personal values when confronted with stories involving moral dilemmas. Brain activity regarding such decisions can be tracked while these people are in the scanner.[42]

Then, of course, there is the most prominent of value-based decisions: "to turn our will and our lives over to God *as we understand Him*" (Step Three). This can clearly be hard to accept for many people. How can such a value-based decision come about?

One way to understand this is to turn to the cognitive dissonance theory, which we discussed in the part of this book related to the AA experience. It posits that people's attitudes can change in a dramatic way when they find themselves having accepted two conflicting positions or sets of values.[43] We had considered this in describing what happens when people experience spiritual awakening, and it can apply to alcoholics who are beginning to buy into AA. They have seen themselves as having had the capacity to drink and not get into trouble, and they forget the times when they would drink uncontrollably.

Classically, the alcoholic in denial says, "I can take it or leave it," believing that he can control his problems. Nonetheless, he is now being pressed to understand that he is "powerless over alcohol" (Step One), and to disavow any such control. This makes for a conflict—a dissonance—between the ideas of self-control and powerlessness. To resolve this, AA provides a dramatically new construct that will relieve this dissonance, namely, that a higher power will govern and guide the addicted person toward an abstinent recovery. This theme certainly runs through the Big Book, and acceptance resolves the problem of the new member's conflicting beliefs: the idea that he can somehow control his drinking versus the acceptance that he has no control. Instead he has a solution: "God as we understood Him" will determine this.

Research into mechanisms underlying the theory of cognitive dissonance is now beginning to clarify the brain sites involved in this process.[44,45] One particular lab study produced dissonance and the need to resolve it. Most people find lying in the fMRI scanner uncomfortable. Research subjects who found it most uncomfortable were told that a very anxious patient, the next person to be scanned, was observing them and their responses behind a one-way mirror in the control room. The subject in the scanner was then asked to respond to sentences they were rating as if they were enjoying the experience. When the ones who showed the biggest change in attitude toward a positive position were scanned, the brain sites that were activated in the face of the dissonance experience were located. Other studies have shown that cognitive dissonance and related activation are associated with negative affect and autonomic arousal, lending emotional weight to the impact of the process.[46] These imaging-based findings pertain to attitudes generated in the laboratory setting, but they do suggest the value of further examination as to how one may accept that a Higher Power can resolve one's conflicting beliefs.

So we end up here with a whole set of recent biological findings that can tie different aspects of the AA experience to specific brain pathways. One can safely say that these are the result of hominid social adaptation and evolution over millennia. Although our conclusions are based on laboratory findings rather than on testing people at AA meetings or while speaking to their sponsors, it certainly suggests that AA's influence is not just that of a bunch of people talking to each other, but rather the engagement of a system that reflects basic neuronal processes, ones that tie in with evolutionary adaptation. The question is whether we can put some of this process to an experimental test.

AN EXPERIMENT

It certainly seemed noteworthy that research findings based on brain imaging might be used to explain how AA members achieve sobriety. This could lend credence to the idea that AA can be seen as a biologically grounded approach to recovery, and could thereby serve as a step toward undertaking more medical research on the fellowship.

Some time after publishing the paper on the work just described, I set up a small meeting of researchers to look at the role of spirituality in AA.

They were drawn from diverse disciplines, from anthropology to neurophysiology. The idea was to develop further our understanding of the many-faceted character of this issue.[47] The meeting also provided a chance to present the model described here and its basis in recent neuroscience research. It was surprising that the members of the group suggested that we should carry out an experimental study at New York University to demonstrate how this actually worked. The idea was appealing, but given the highly technical nature of any fMRI research, it was clearly beyond the technical capacity of my group to undertake.

After reflecting on how such a study could be helpful in getting through to the biologically oriented academic medical community, and after considering my foray into studying the world of fMRI, I looked into the research areas pursued by senior NYU faculty who were involved with imaging research. Although their expertise could probably be applied to such a study, none seemed to be involved in work that related to a topic like AA, and certainly not in work related to the role of a higher power in one's life.

I asked further, and in the end, I was told of a junior faculty member, Zoran Josipovic, who had studied the effect of Buddhist meditation on the brain. Zoran was well aware of the pressure that senior research scientists experienced in assuring continuation in their government-funded research. He also was aware that the NIH peer groups who passed on grant applications might look askance on an investigator who had anything to do with spirituality, or even with a successful fellowship like AA. They would likely be viewed as flighty by some reviewers who took a dim view of anything to do with the role of religion in contemporary life.

The culture of the NIH grant reviews is relevant here. Thomas Kuhn, you may recall, spoke of normal science, the way researchers come to look at the phenomena they are studying at a given time, and how they may become bound to particular research paradigms.[48] This means, in effect, that other approaches to study may seem to be inappropriate for research. The NIH review committees, although composed of highly respected scientists, stick closely to the established empirical paradigms with which they are familiar. They also operate in a climate where funding is so tight that even one member of a review committee questioning an applicant's work could score their proposal low enough to leave it unfunded. The senior NYU researchers would not want any aspect of their efforts to become controversial in such a climate.

So we decided to go ahead with the project outside the NIH system. The funds I had on hand for such a project from ongoing support from the John

Templeton Foundation were limited, but Templeton had a history of interest in research related to spirituality, so it was OK to use them for this purpose.

Our previous experience with long-term AA members was that many were willing to commit time and effort to a project they thought could ultimately benefit other alcoholics, and we had contact information for many of them. We had no funds to pay them to participate in an elaborate fMRI protocol, and it was not likely that they would be interested in committing themselves to such a project for modest financial compensation; the mission of AA members was to "give back" for the recovery they had been offered by the program. Their interest was not pecuniary.

I considered two options for adapting previous imaging studies to develop our protocol. One was to make use of members' fidelity to the fellowship's mission of aiding alcoholic people in distress. We could compare their response to images of distressed alcoholic people to that of persons who had no alcohol problems. This would test the edict of "carrying the message to other alcoholics." We would draw on the experience of a published study[49] I had described here, which had distinguished the responses of subjects coming to the aid of people on a soccer team they root for, as compared to coming to the aid of members of an opposing team.

Another option was to consider an aspect of AA ritual to see if it could generate a decrease in alcohol-related craving when members were exposed to alcohol triggers. This latter option was more appealing because it went to the heart of the AA regimen and belief in a higher power. Our hypothesis would be that long-term abstinent AA members exposed to alcohol triggers could avoid a craving response when they drew on such AA practices. An explicit AA ritual that we could apply in the scanner was that of the recitation of AA prayers. After all, Step Eleven reads, "Sought through prayer and meditation to improve our conscious connection with God, *as we understood Him. . . .*"

I had been struck by how committed AA members could draw on prayer to bolster their sobriety in the face of triggering circumstances. One member had told me of a time that she had volunteered to participate in an addiction study at the imaging center at Brookhaven National Laboratories on Long Island. She said that she was worried that the drug-related imagery they would show her might lead her to be vulnerable to relapse. She said that she had recited AA prayers to fortify herself on the train ride all the way to the lab.

Bill C, who had been an invaluable liaison to fellowship members, pointed out two prayers that were spelled out in the Big Book, one on Step Three, and the other on Step Seven. The Step Three prayer, and the now famous Serenity Prayer, seemed like good candidates for use in the study.

The former was rather formulaic. It runs like this: "God, I offer myself to Thee—to build with me and to do with me as Thou wilt. Relieve me of the bondage of self. . . ."[50] The Serenity Prayer has long been associated with AA, although it is well-known to the general public: "God, grant me the serenity to accept the things that I cannot change; the courage to change the things I can, and the wisdom to know the difference."

Our protocol[51] involved having the subjects briefed on the procedures we would carry out and then to have them give formal consent in line with NYU's requirements for research on human subjects. (This employs elaborate documents, grown more so over time to prevent any mistreatment of people in medical research.) They provided us background information with a survey instrument like the ones we had used in our studies of Young People in AA and Doctors in AA. After that, we had them lie down in the scanner. The key element in the study was for them to be presented, while in the scanner, with pictures of alcoholic drinks or of people drinking. These presentations were applied under each of two different conditions: after reading neutral material drawn from a newspaper and, separately, after reciting the AA prayers. Our plan was to see if the subjects reported greater craving after the neutral material than after the prayers. That is to say, did praying decrease their craving, and hence their vulnerability to drinking? If so, we would examine whether the scanner had picked up on what was going on in the brain while this was happening.

Getting the necessary number of volunteers, many of whom had to travel over an hour each way to the scanning lab, took some time. The twenty who did come were quite cooperative and willing to lie still in the scanner for over an hour without moving, while the whole detailed protocol played out. This was no small matter, because lying still in a scanner for that long a time is not pleasant.

I had framed an accompanying survey instrument along with Helen Dermatis, a colleague in my Division. Details on the scanning procedure, the programming needed to run the protocol in the scanner, and analysis of the data emerging were technically quite complex. This was being framed by Zoran and Helen with consultation from colleagues of Zoran's at Columbia and Yale.

The results were quite telling. Subjects reported that they experienced little or no craving in their daily routines during the previous week. When shown the trigger pictures, though, they did report some low-grade craving. Interestingly, their craving did not show up in the brain site called the striatum, where it typically would in detoxified alcoholic patients. It appeared that the craving may have emanated from some other process. It would be revealing to figure this out.

The effect that AA prayer had on the brain helped to explain this. When subjects read the prayers, they felt less craving than when they read neutral material. This decrease in craving after prayer was associated with brain areas that regulate self-control and interpret the meaning of the outside stimuli. Apparently these made for the unconscious neural process that the prayers could induce, which served to modify what the trigger pictures elicited.

It appears that the experience of AA over the years had left these fellowship members with an innate ability to use the AA experience— prayer in the case of this study—to minimize the effect of alcohol triggers in producing craving. This was done without them actively exerting themselves. One might say that the AA experience had created a new understanding of themselves relative to their old addict self, that is, a new self-schema. This new self-schema was effectively one of a person who does not crave alcohol in the face of temptation. The self-schema does this implicitly by summoning up their neural armaments against temptation.

So from where did the modest level of craving emanate when it showed up long after people had stopped drinking? Because it did not appear to come from the striatum, where changes were shown in recently detoxified alcoholics, perhaps it was actually a learned emotional response to triggers. I thought of the way a patient of mine, who had long suffered from severe depression, and then recovered with proper support and therapy, would interpret subtle mood fluctuations as a potential recurrence of depression, even though he was, in fact, not relapsing into his depressive illness. Over the years he had "learned" to associate these modest depressive triggers with the idea of depressive illness, whereas people who had never suffered a depressive illness would not perceive them that way. In this way, a conditioned feeling of craving may represent a lingering vulnerability to relapse. Triggers summon up this "learned" feeling of craving in folks who had lots of prior experience with craving before they had acquired an innate protection against it.

SOME OBSERVATIONS

This model on long-term recovery is compatible with some aspects of addiction that seem counterintuitive. One is its puzzling nature as an illness vulnerable to relapse: Why is it that an alcoholic can suddenly fall back into drinking, even after years of sobriety? Here is another aspect of the disease that is hard to explain: Why is it that some people can stay in AA and go to meetings for years, and still be pressured by craving for alcohol? Many people who qualify speak to their fellow members, saying, "It's a struggle every day."

Let's consider these questions by recourse to the fMRI research I reviewed and what we found in our study. Our subjects had all reported having had a spiritual awakening and were comfortably abstinent. We could surmise that they had been transformed from a self-schema of someone who needs a drink—who struggles with the conditioned feeling of craving—to a new self-schema of someone who has the innate capacity to control and delimit attention to craving. This may have happened dramatically in their spiritual awakening, or it may have come about gradually. Either way, it yields a limited responsiveness to alcohol triggers. This is why such long-term members can pass by liquor stores on the way home from work unperturbed, or encounter the upsetting vagaries of life without relapsing. And it is also seems evident that their AA prayers can bolster this transformed state.

We can consider another aspect of relapse in alcohol addiction. Alcoholics who apparently have achieved a long-term stable sobriety can relapse as well, particularly if for some reason they have an unsettling disappointment that moves them to take a drink. Why might an initial lapse after one drink or two lead them to "going out," as they say, being pulled back into a period of heavy bingeing, just as they had been doing before becoming committed to recovery? Perhaps the disruption of having a modest lapse to alcohol can lead to the re-emergence of the drinking self-schema, which had been submerged for a time, perhaps even a long time. The noncraving sense of self, whose acquired mechanisms divert responsivity to alcohol triggers, is superseded by an earlier compulsive self, which was present in dormant form.

We may draw on a phenomenon described by research psychologists to explain how previously extinguished habits (conditioned responses) can later re-emerge. Coincidently, they call this spontaneous recovery, but they are not referring to the kind of recovery we mean in AA terms. What applies here is that old habits, which were superseded by new ones, can re-emerge, that is to say, be spontaneously recovered from the past. Similarly, a new memory can be superseded by the one thought to have been superseded originally.[52] Such events are particularly more likely to occur if one returns to the context where the old memory or habit had been established.[53] This could be a physical setting (a bar) or an emotional setting (depressing circumstances).

To clarify further, we can hark back to the model of classical conditioning described earlier. One primary characteristic of addictive drugs is the following: When a person is dosed with an addictive agent for a period of time, their body reacts with an opposite response, like a withdrawal reaction, effectively stabilizing itself. The response to alcohol, an agent that depresses consciousness, breathing, and the like, is countered by activating a withdrawal agitation—which can show up as malaise or tremor. This adaptive response is characteristic of drugs that are addictive. Another example: Cocaine, a stimulant, induces an opposite depressive reaction that is seen after one "crashes," becomes depressed, after a cocaine binge.

So a reactive agitation, or similar emotional pressure underlying heavy drinking, can take place in triggering settings, ones that had been regularly paired with drinking before the person achieved sobriety. It becomes a conditioned—a habituated—response. For example, the innate response of agitation in response to alcohol may have been paired many times with being in a bar or getting depressed. Like Pavlov's dogs, the pairing of an innate withdrawal response with triggering stimuli can break through a sober self-schema that one had acquired as one who craves no more, leaving the drinker vulnerable to conditioned craving and alcohol-seeking. The old schema is, as we just mentioned, recovered, that is, comes out again. A recovering alcoholic might have drunk whenever he got depressed, so he might be vulnerable to reactive craving if he got depressed, even after he had been abstinent for a long time. And hence, a potential relapse.

FOR EACH PERSON, PRAYER HAS ITS OWN CHARACTER

Let's not forget that we were dealing with real people in our study, not just faceless volunteers. This is important because one of the prayers that we used in our study was spelled out in the Big Book, the Third Step Prayer. The other, the Serenity prayer, is widely available. But over the years of membership, our participants had tailored their prayers to their own personal inclinations and needs. In fact, the individual nature of these choices reflects how personalized the AA experience can be for each respective member. It shows how any attempt to generalize either subjective or neural aspects of prayer cannot fully capture prayer's complex and personal nature for a given member. We have to accept this limitation and, for that matter, the limits on generalizing any aspect of addiction recovery across the board.

This limitation certainly applied to the framing of our protocol. The key element in the study was to determine the impact of prayer on a subject's response to alcohol-trigger images. We had the subjects read the two prayers, which were familiar to them. Would they have responded to prayers of their own choice with an even greater effect? My guess is that if each subject could have chosen a particular prayer, the impact would have been greater. In that case, though, the project would have been open to question as to whether there was consistency in the very variable that we were studying. A research project inevitably requires a certain rigidity in structure, which may remove it from the realities of "real" life.

Helen Dermatis, Ali Millard, and I reviewed interviews with our participants in the fMRI study, and we saw various aspects of the prayer experience in how they described their own use of this ritual. It is important to note that these members are among the most committed. Although they are influential in transmitting the culture of the fellowship, the depth of their prayer does not necessarily reflect that of newer members.

The content of the prayer could vary from time to time, but it generally related to communication with an actual deity, albeit one without a specific identity. Here are some examples of what the participants reported.

Prayer can be confined to a particular time or place, like morning or evening, but it also can take place at other times of day, such as here:

> Prayer is about communication with the Higher Power, more of a talking-to. And you want to know how I do it? There is a formal practice that I do in the morning and sometimes at night. Then there is intermittent communication that I do throughout the day, like when I am driving or working, when it's not a verbal communication but a mental communication.

This fits in well with the reports of many of the longtime members: They were in God's presence every day, even all day. So why not turn to him at different times; he is an available source of comfort and well-being that one can rely on for emotional support when feeling a need, even for momentary relief or companionship from this all-knowing benign figure. The encounters can be almost conversational:

> I consider prayer to be a petition that I am saying to my Higher Power whom I call God. It's like me saying, "I am here, God. I know you're there too and I know you are watching over me and that I am in good times." I always feel comfortable when I do that, when I acknowledge that there is a power greater than myself who certainly helps me stay sober on a daily basis, but also in my day-to-day life as well.

Early in sobriety, on the other hand, prayer typically relates to a new member's need to avoid a return to drinking ("going out"), and it can be learned by example from another member.

> In the very beginning, I only had two weeks [of sobriety] and someone else had three weeks, and I was like, "How did you do that?" And he told me that he prayed. I thought he was pulling my leg. The next morning I got up and got on my knees and I prayed with all of my heart. It was the first time in twenty years. I really asked to not go out that day.

The charismatic gift of access to God is transmitted from one generation of members to the next. It allows for a transformative experience, just as Bill W had in AA's seminal moment with his "white light" experience.

Prayer practice does evolve over time. It can include specific text from the Big Book, but it need not be defined in that way, and it can be personally conceived.

> My definition of prayer is open-ended. It's pretty much ever-evolving, only I don't know what it will be when it changes and what it will change to. There have been periods of my life when I use the written word, whether it be from the religion that I come from or from the literature of AA. There have been times when I have used sounds like chanting, just going with the spirit of intention more than language.

As members begin to move toward an awakening, or after having had such an experience, they act on the flexibility accorded them in the fellowship to worship as they choose. There is no catechism that would dictate doctrine for proper worship, as in an orthodox system of Christian belief.

For one of our subjects, with no religious inclination, the prayer experience was rather vague, more of an emotional state:

> I usually do it in the mornings, sometimes at night or throughout the day. It means talking to or connecting with some sort of spirituality or higher power or force. I think it is important and it is something that means a lot to me even though it is hard to describe and put a finger on, but it represents my emotional state and my emotional being and comfort, maturity, growth, all of those things.

In Step Eleven, members avow that they have "sought through prayer and meditation" to come closer to their Higher Power, so a certain obligation is implied. Even someone who is not inclined toward prayer will feel the need to fulfill this, however diffuse their own practice of it may be.

One's higher power need not be an externally perceived entity. One can experience the God to whom one prays as residing within oneself, reflecting "feeling God's presence" every day.

> When you say AA prayer it sounds as if it is a specific thing. I have now grown in AA to the point where I have a much better understanding of my God, the God within me. I think it is all within me. It's not outside of me, it's all inside of me.

We were particularly interested in the study participants' use of the Serenity Prayer, given that we had employed it in our own study. Respondents could express it explicitly as a prayer, or it could be used as a guiding philosophy for dealing with what life doles out.

> The Serenity Prayer. I utilized that in the beginning. It was constantly, every day. Sometimes I needed that to be going through my mind every waking moment in my thoughts, as I was doing things. I was using that prayer to help me get through the day and to not want to pick up that drink . . . So when I was in my work environment and I was around people who don't have the program that I have been blessed with, there are a lot of occasions when I needed to just step aside and ask God to help me work with this person, or I prayed for this person with the Serenity prayer to help me get through that moment.

This suggests that prayer can help to assure emotional stability, or help to maintain a character that one sees to be worthy of an AA member. This was described by two of the participants in our study:

> In the Third Step Prayer, there are three promises. "Relieve me of the bondage of self, so that I may better do Thy will" is one of them. So I say that prayer when I feel bonded to self, which can take a number of forms: mental constriction, depression, or anger.
>
> I kind of do it preventatively now. In the very beginning I would "white knuckle" it: Oh God, please get me through this, help me out just one day at a time. But today I don't have that. Right now in my life there is a little more self-reproachment happening. I pray to not get too cocky. I am afraid if I get cocky I might go out. But I don't get those urges right now.

Prayer can then be a mantra to help maintain an admirable character, or even serve as a bulwark against the distress that patients turning to therapy might otherwise encounter. The mutuality and social support in the fellowship are supposed to help people act with the integrity associated with Twelve Step recovery. They can, with prayer as an accompanying practice, also help to stabilize a person with mental illness.

Prayer can be an aid to sobriety, but it is often directed to the benefit of others, to play a role in AA's expectation of service to other alcoholics. It can bind a person to all members of the fellowship, even worldwide:

> There are times that I've done service, now that I am thinking about it, that it feels like an extension of prayer. I get to be a part of someone's life in an active way, a positive way. . . . I can pray for people that are in the fellowship that I may or may not know, so that connects me to them as well.

For some, it can certainly relate to their traditional religious background.

> I was afraid to go back to Church because I didn't want them to tell me that I was doing something wrong. But I met a woman in one of the groups who felt the same way I did, and who also practiced the same religion I did, and she also wanted to go back to Church. So you know, God writes straight with crooked lines, we went back to church together and we learned together to take what we need and leave the rest behind.

Our participants were drawn from the New York area, and their ties to church-based religious practice was likely to be less, on average, than might be the case in some other areas of the country. Most did not report that their prayers were closely tied to a specific denomination, or its respective rituals. In communities where ties to a church or parish are more common, their description of prayers would likely be more in line with traditional congregational practices. The fact that most of our participants' prayers did not relate to the God of a particular denomination, however, did not apparently dampen their commitment to the higher power to which they could relate. They all saw such commitment as compelling in guiding the course of their lives.

One might be impressed that AA apparently "trains" the brain to carry out its lessons. Presumably, it does this by reinterpreting the impact of alcohol-related triggers in the environment, and thereby helping members exercise control over them. And AA prayer epitomizes this. This lends credence to the fact that AA represents more than a group of people talking and sharing. Instead, the fellowship experience seems to provide neurally based means for transforming people's innate sense of self—their self-schema—into a sober one, thereby changing the way they perceive the world of drinking triggers they encounter. If such findings can be expanded on, we may gain a better understanding about the nature of long-term recovery for AA members, and perhaps as well for people who achieve long-term recovery by other means.

CHAPTER 12

Alcoholics Anonymous's Effectiveness

Nowadays, physicians, insurers, and the federal government regard "evidence-based medicine" as essential in determining how illnesses should be treated. "Evidence-based" is a term that originated in the 1980s from the work of David Eddy, a physician and mathematician at Stanford University. The idea behind it lay in the observation that there were wide variations in the way physicians practiced; many of the procedures that they applied were considered ill-advised even among their expert colleagues.

Eddy avowed that medical practice should be based on demonstrated scientific findings, and we now have come to see randomized controlled trials (RCTs) as the best basis for such findings: Treatments should be subjected to evaluation by comparing them to alternative options under well-delineated conditions, and with the assignment of patients at random to either the approach to be tested or to a comparison treatment option. Interestingly, we now see articles in major publications like the *Journal of the American Medical Association* reflecting negative results about treatment approaches that have been undertaken for some time based on what was thought to be good clinical judgment.

But the reality is that much of what physicians do from day to day is not easily subjected to RCTs. What is more, in the domain of addiction treatment, we have almost no systematic findings on the long-term outcome of our interventions, even if they were subjected to RCTs. The outcomes of federal and drug company studies often are measured only in terms of weeks, certainly not years. Do these treatments have a material impact in the long term? We have little if any research in this domain. Furthermore, the actual results of an intervention in "real life," called ecologic validity, can be very different from when the intervention is applied in an RCT protocol with patients being monitored by research staff on a regular basis. An example of this might be seen in the findings of the federal Project MATCH, a study we will discuss shortly, whose data are widely cited by researchers. Little if any difference was found in comparing an AA-based approach to two other modalities. The elaborate nature of the monitoring and testing of subjects in this study may have gotten them to keep their drinking in line as much as the treatments themselves. After all, the researchers were dealing with a disease where a person's attitude influences the outcome. All the subjects got a very clear message from the overall protocol that they were supposed to overcome their drinking problems, and were monitored over the course of the study to see how they "performed." Such oversight could even have as much influence as the treatments being tested.

In the popular media, AA is the remedy that gets mentioned most often for alcohol and other drug problems, but many doctors and patients are aware that questions are being raised these days about its effectiveness. Some critiques are posed by people who give anecdotal evidence of problems associated with AA, or by people who have not benefited from the fellowship and have turned elsewhere. These detractors range from journalists who claim that the Twelve Step approach is outdated and ineffective,[1] to some psychiatrists who assume that alcoholic patients can be treated by psychotherapy alone.[2] Speculative, even dubious approaches, like equine therapy, health food fads, and the like, which are touted in some rehabs, may be included among the questionable practices cited, even though they have nothing to do with AA as such. Then there are research-based clinical scientists who point to studies that examine alternative approaches for treatments based on medications, some quite effective, others less so.[3,4] These approaches may, in fact, be compatible with AA, and they can be used by an addiction professional in conjunction with referral to a Twelve Step program.

STUDYING THE OUTCOME OF AA

So how well *does* AA work? This is a question with no easy answer. It is like the question a parent may ask when bringing an adolescent substance abuser to me for treatment: "How will my son do?" In such cases, I try to be encouraging to the extent appropriate, but point out that every person is particular, and the way treatment will unfold depends on their own unique circumstances. An experienced clinician can surmise, but only surmise, how a given patient will do in the long term.

Given the widespread use of AA among addicted people and the need to understand its overall effectiveness, the outcome for alcoholic people who are exposed to it has, indeed, been the subject of some very thoughtfully conducted research. These studies, however, inevitably suffer from a very telling limitation: AA is not like a pill given for an illness in general medicine, to be taken for an easily defined syndrome, like penicillin for pneumococcal pneumonia. Alcohol presents different faces in different people, and it evokes different experiences depending on the person's social environment, as well as her or his genetics. Furthermore, AA is not a "treatment" as such. It is best approached along with help from an addiction professional, and the relationship between the treater and patient, relative to how the referral is proposed, can be crucial to whether the patient will attend and respond positively.

An approach for how professionals can promote a patient's involvement in AA has been thoughtfully developed, and spelled out by expert clinical researchers, and it has been shown to enhance the likelihood that someone will successfully engage in the fellowship. Called Twelve Step Facilitation (TSF),[5] it was designed to be applied over twelve sessions, two of which can include the patient's spouse. Patients are encouraged to go to several AA meetings a week, read the AA Big Book, and to not drink at all. Sessions focus on understanding and accepting the first three Steps of AA to the extent that the patient can. In Project Match,[6] this approach worked well compared to two other professional modalities (cognitive behavioral therapy and motivational enhancement). Each of the three approaches was found suitable to the variety of patients with whom it was applied. TSF, though, was found to be relatively more effective for people who were embedded in social networks of family or friends who were heavy drinkers.[7]

Researchers who want to study AA's effectiveness are restricted by the limitations spelled out in AA's Traditions. These include anonymity among AA's members, no affiliation with outside organizations, and the fact that local groups are not obliged to cooperate with AA's General Service Board. There are, however, studies by leading researchers like John Kelly[8,9] that have shed light on AA's effectiveness overall. And "overall" is a key word here, because, as I pointed out, each alcoholic is a unique case of his or her own. The most recent compendium of technically grounded research that one might want to turn to is available in a volume that I coedited with Lee Ann Kaskutas reviewing hundreds of published studies on AA research.[10]

Dr. Kaskutas, however, wrote one review of how epidemiological criteria can be applied successfully to the studies that are available to test whether AA can be considered effective.[11] The approach she used was first introduced to assist policymakers in evaluating causality in relation to whether smoking was related to lung cancer.[12] There, too, randomized controlled trials were not possible; one could not assign half of a group of teenagers to smoke for thirty years and the others to never smoke at all, just as no one can make one group of people go to AA and tell another group that they cannot go to AA.

Two of the points she made are worth noting. A medicine's effectiveness often is judged by whether there is a relationship between the dose given and the degree to which it relieves the symptoms of the illness being treated. She pointed to a study[13] that found that abstinence rates a year after treatment were directly correlated with how many Twelve Step meetings the addicted person had attended that year. Secondly, she pointed out that the fellowship's causal relationship to improvement was supported by the fact that AA attendance was found to *precede* subsequent abstinence in both untreated[14] and treated[15] alcoholics, rather than follow it.

A question remains, though: Do the people who chose to go to AA just have the makeup, in some way unknown to researchers, to become abstinent more than those who keep drinking? This would make AA's outcome look better simply because the AA attenders were more likely to stay abstinent, regardless of whether they went to the program. So how can one get around this potential bias? In order to deal with this, Keith Humphreys and colleagues considered an ingenious way of analyzing available data on AA outcomes.[16] They found studies where people were assigned at random to TSF as compared to those who were given other treatments. Inevitably, some people in the non-TSF condition chose to go to AA, regardless of how they were assigned, and the research group counted them separately. The researchers were then able to isolate results of the people who went to AA versus those who did not, independent of their own prior preference, thereby avoiding the criticism leveled on AA outcome studies that people who chose to go to AA were the ones more open to improvement. And this did imply that AA benefited the people in the study independent of whatever their prior likelihood for abstinence might be.

On the other hand, there is one characteristic that is most likely to lead one alcoholic rather than another to join AA, namely the greater severity of his or her problem.[17] This can be understood from the observation that George Vaillant, a leader in framing our understanding of alcoholism, made in his book, *The Natural History of Alcoholism*.[18] The more severe a person's alcohol problem, the less likely he is to achieve stability unless he stops drinking completely. Once a person has reached the level where an alcohol problem has become an addiction, controlled drinking rarely presents a viable option.

Vaillant saw alcoholism as an illness vulnerable to yielding repeated relapses. So it makes sense that AA, with its emphasis on permanent abstinence, is a likelier fit for the more severe alcoholic. It makes a resource like AA, which is available for one to turn to as needed, so useful. We see apparent examples of this severity issue throughout this book. The most committed long-term members—and the ones who went on to spiritual awakening—told their stories in terms of the profound disruption and despair they had experienced. Just like the alcoholics portrayed in the movies I described, many of these are people whose problems are not likely to be modified without something as compelling as Twelve Step renewal.

One more study: How well do women do in AA? This is interesting because at its inception, the fellowship was restricted to men only. Also, one might think that women would be less comfortable in AA, given that they might be reluctant to be seen as tainted by addiction. It turned out that when alcoholic people receiving treatment were followed up three years after treatment, the likelihood of being abstinent in AA was significantly greater for women than men, and women had a better overall outcome as well.[19]

So how do I—and how do you, the reader—make sense of the question, "Does AA work for a given person?" In the first place, it has been found that once people have sought out treatment for alcoholism, a majority of them will go to AA.[20, 21] For alcoholic people seeking help, both AA participation alone or formal treatment alone were associated with an improved outcome.[22] Those with the best outcome, however, had both AA and treatment.[23]

How about initial motivation? One study, which measured how motivated patients were at the outset of treatment, was particularly telling. It might seem that those who were most open to dealing with their drinking problem would be the ones who would get involved in AA. It turns out that the greater likelihood of doing better did not depend on how motivated a patient had been when treatment began.[24] So it appears that, across the board, AA attendance after professional treatment is associated with improved outcome independent of a person's prior motivation.

These are only findings across the board, as they apply to large numbers of patients on average. Much of an expert clinician's judgment regarding a given patient has to rest on the variety of experiences the clinician has had with patients, because each patient has her own universe of circumstances. So, I thought it would be useful to give the reader some examples to illustrate the diverse issues that impact on different patients in relation to AA. This way you can get an idea of what can come to bear on the outcome of the AA encounter in given individuals.

A certain portion of members follow the full, traditional sequence of joining:

Ali did well in business school in London, got a job in banking in the States, and married a woman from Amman who had been his sweetheart. His drinking, though, was getting worse over the ten years before I saw him. He was passing out asleep now every evening, and had moved from job to job related to instability secondary to his drinking problem, much to the distress of his wife. As we began treatment, Ali agreed to go to AA meetings to see if they were right for him. He soon started attending on a regular basis. He found the time spent there comforting, clearly it seemed, because of the atmosphere of unconditional acceptance he encountered. I also prescribed medication for him that is associated with his alcohol craving, along with a medication for his apparent social anxiety. He stopped drinking after we first met.

I met with Ali and his wife a number of times, and she complained that he tended to isolate himself, even when he was now sober, and she felt a gulf between them when they were at home together. His isolation was evident in his spending time on his computer rather than socializing with her, and was also evident when they had gone to spend time with her family in Jordan. Ali and I discussed how this was related to an anxiety disorder along with social anxiety he had suffered from for many years. The difficulty also derived from an abusive relationship he had experienced at the hands of his father, who had been derisive of him, particularly when the Dad himself was drinking heavily.

On a number of occasions Ali would mention his comfort in going to the AA meetings, and it was clear that in his case, the feeling of acceptance among the members gave him relief from the isolation and malaise that had characterized his relationships over many years. Nonetheless, even after most of the anxiety had abated, I had to take time to help him to understand why his inclination to isolate himself was a habit that could be broken.

After two months in AA he had acquired a sponsor and began working the Steps. He brought his wife to some AA meetings and to social events held by some longstanding members, and also went with other members to a twelve-session Big Book course to review the text in detail. His vulnerability to guilt, however, came up in dealing with the working of Step Four, "making a searching and fearless moral inventory," and again on Step Nine, "making amends." It related to an experience of his while still in college in Jordan. As a student, he had worked in sales in a small appliance store, where he had been manipulated and underpaid by the owner. On one occasion, he had pilfered a small amount of cash from the till, and now felt obliged to make amends for this, but since the owner was no longer available to him, he found this gap in his Step work upsetting. He pondered this in one session:

> I can't call and make the amends. So the question is, where am I standing with the Steps? I'm constantly questioning if I have done it well enough. But then comes the question, compared to what? Based on what? Is it three out of ten? But what's ten and what's three? That's why probably I need help.

It was only with difficulty that his sponsor, and I as well, could help him come to terms with the fact that he could be absolved of the obligation to make amends for the deed.

After two years, Ali told a meeting chair that he was willing to take on a sponsee. His involvement in the program was now notable in how well he adapted to it despite his initial guilt over Step Nine. Only on rare occasions did he report that a disruptive experience would lead to some minor cravings.

WHEN GOING "LITE" WAS EASY

Not all involvements in AA follow the full-fledged course of the program. Sam had a successful experience in therapy combined with a limited exposure to AA. Both were positive for him, and worked in concert to help him stop drinking. This is an example of how AA can be helpful even if it does not involve going through all its rituals.

Susie, Sam's wife, was chronically depressed and always angry at him because he drank too much. In addition to ending his evenings at home by falling asleep after his regular heavy drinking, he had embarrassed her on many occasions, having noticeably been drinking heavily when they were out to dinner with friends. She told him that he had to deal with his problem, and her psychiatrist referred him to me.

Sam was in the doghouse. Susie did not let him sleep in their bedroom. She confronted him over his two teenage daughters' view of him as less of a father than they wanted. He was derided for being guilty of a DWI (a citation for driving while intoxicated) that had led to a six-month suspension of his driver's license. Like many people with moderate but not the most severe of problems, he did not, however, overtly compromise his career, as he never drank excessively during business events.

Sam showed up in therapy as an engaging and talkative fellow. He was willing to follow the recommendation I made that there was little benefit with just moderating his drinking. Better to stop. Additionally, since he was annoyed at his wife's chronic irritability, he thought there was a good reason to set an example of abstinence for her.

Sam had always seen himself as limited in what he could accomplish in life. His father had demeaned him while idealizing his older brother. He underperformed at school while the brother applied himself diligently and excelled. He allowed himself to be berated by his wife for any failings of his own, which, even if real, were not deserving of her boisterous and derisive behavior. At work, the manager of his firm regularly disparaged him, but he had tolerated this for over a decade when he could have sought out more promising opportunities. Our attention to improving these situations was reassuring to him, and over the course of treatment he came to realize that he was not destined for—nor did he have to accept—the harsh treatment directed at him. His experience in AA was positive as well, albeit relatively limited. He began attending, initially with some reluctance, but soon accommodated himself to going twice weekly. As he was sociable by nature, he was comfortable sharing at meetings.

After some time, I asked him about the one meeting he went to where everyone was expected to speak. What did he do there?

I definitely share about having a fucked up boss, and being in a tremendously toxic work situation. I might share about my father, who is eighty-nine and just broke his hip, and has been in the hospital a couple of times. I might give a two-minute speech about how my brother isn't doing anything for him and how it upsets me, and how I have to deal with this, and it's very difficult. Inevitably, it could possibly be something about Susie, too. But I inevitably find that there is someone there who is in their mid-fifties, or whose father has just died, or aunt or mother is sick, or mother-in-law. Everybody deals with the same thing, and its good feedback to hear that I am not the only one.

Do you talk about your Higher Power?

I might say something like I'm not a religious guy. I'm certainly not going to talk about religion at a meeting because they don't really want to hear that. But I might say that an understanding of God in my own way has been very helpful to me. Why do I have to say more? I might just say that.

Do you have any established relationships with people there?

Yes, I know a lot of people that I say hello to and talk to a little bit.

Like how much?

How much do I talk to them? Like do I spend an hour afterwards? No.

What do you say?

I might say, "How are you doing?" In other words, not a real conversation, but mutual recognition and part of a social milieu, without being in active exchange with people, so to speak. I might say, "How's your week?" Someone might have heard me the week before if I went back to the same meeting, and asked, "How'd it go this week with your father?"

What happened with sponsorship?

Nothing.

Sam continued to attend over the course of the year that we met, and for some months thereafter. Some time later he had occasion to see me, and he still acknowledged that his best course was to maintain abstinence, and he had had no episodes of drinking.

How did AA help him? Was it necessary? I think it was valuable in helping him identify with the culture of abstinence, so that he became comfortable with not drinking when he was at social occasions, and stopped drinking at home. There was one time while we were meeting that a glass of wine was poured for him while he was at a dinner with other couples, and he unthinkingly took a sip, and then pulled back feeling very remorseful. An episode like this showed how AA had helped him by fortifying his abstinence. By the way, his wife came to be more positively disposed toward him and came to seek out his advice and support.

WHEN MOTIVATION TO JOIN AA COMES ABOUT INADVERTENTLY

At first glance, it would seem that most people who decide on their own to go to AA do so because drinking or drugs were potentially bringing ruin upon them. They do not quite know where else to turn, and AA is readily available to anyone almost anywhere. We know from research that most people derive some benefit if referred in a systematic way by a treatment program. But what about those people who start going without a professional referral? Ron's experience reflects that many people go for reasons that do not show up in statistics, and end up turning to AA almost unexpectedly.

Ron had originally come to see me because of his concern over his son's cocaine addiction. We both spoke with the son, who was reluctant to lend any credence to what we were offering. I was puzzled. The son's despair— he was in debt, increasingly isolated, and about to be fired from his job— would be the basis for many patients' accepting help in such an encounter. He seemed to have some other reason for refusing.

I called Ron two years later to follow up on the mystery. His son eventually did go to the rehab program that I had recommended, but it was only when we spoke this second time that Ron acknowledged his own heavy drinking to me, at least a pint of vodka every night. This had clearly compromised the credibility of our discussion with his son. He then told me how he himself found his way to AA and how it opened a door to him for spiritual renewal:

It was my son's first week at the rehab and I was at a family meeting, a very emotional meeting. They asked everyone to say something and all I could say was, "I should be in AA, too," and a few days later I went to my first meeting.

And how did you get involved in AA's spirituality?

I wasn't a religious man, and when I first entered the program, for the first few months I couldn't make sense of a Higher Power, so for me the Higher Power was the group. I wasn't sure how to relate to the program, and my concept of God was lost long ago from my Jewish background. But then I began reading a page or two of AA's daily reflections and then a page or two from the book a rabbi wrote about AA. It took me a year and a half until I began to understand the concept of a Higher Power. And then the God of my understanding became *Hashem* [Hebrew for the deity].

Ron had felt guilty over his role in his son's refusal of treatment, and it had driven him to spontaneously confess his alcoholism at the hospital's family meeting. He knew that he had been living a lie, one that might have cost his son dearly. He had apparently felt like a sinner, much like a person who is driven to go up front at a religious revival meeting, begging Jesus for forgiveness.

WHITE KNUCKLING IT

AA can hardly overcome adverse events that are so compelling that they cast a spell over the struggle for recovery. Here is what these events were in Carl's case: A severe injury that ended his career and crippled his pride; resentment over being forced to do housework and cater to his working wife; his wife's simmering anger and attacks over his history of addiction; siblings who drank heavily and derided him for his abstinence.

Carl had been a successful sales executive who could always socialize while drinking heavily along with his brothers or with clients. At the age of forty, an auto accident left him wheelchair-bound and supported full-time by his firm's disability insurance. With little feeling of autonomy and with despair over his limitations, he fell into a pattern of compulsive drinking. While he was drinking to excess, his wife Liz's career took off, but the demands of her work kept her at the beck and call of her law firm at all hours, and on weekends, too. Carl grew bitter over his career of babysitting their six-year-old, doing the wash, and preparing dinner for his wife. He ended up in rehab, and upon leaving he was ambivalent about abstinence. Although he was attending AA, it was a struggle for him every day to avoid going out to drink. He tried hard, but could not move beyond his bitterness and "white knuckling" his sobriety.

Relapse ensued, and he ended up back in rehab. After his discharge, Liz was unable to reconcile herself to her onerous work schedule and the cost of her husband's rehabs. She began to let out her frustration by yelling at him, and blaming him for what she saw as his ruining both their lives and endangering their child.

When I first saw Carl he was an embittered man, under siege, reluctantly attending an evening group-treatment program, and going to AA intermittently. He spoke to me of the burden of anger he felt, having to stay sober and being subject to diatribes from his wife, including her constantly pressing him on whether he had again begun drinking. I asked what the relapse that brought him to rehab was like:

Do you remember fighting with Liz so you could go and buy liquor?
Yeah. I told her to get away from me. I said, 'Don't you dare follow me.' I said, 'What are you doing?' She thinks that she's my mother.
Well, she was trying to keep you from destroying yourself. You have to distinguish between Liz trying to save your life and her being annoying.
Yes, and when I'm perfectly sober I totally understand that. But in that situation I was insane. When she follows me around like that it's not good. There'd never be a good outcome.
You were drunk. You were driving your son crazy; you were injuring yourself. She was trying to keep you from killing yourself. Are you blaming her for that?
No, I'm not blaming her for that. When I'm in the height of my addiction, it's sick, because I can't control it. Because when she's on me

like that, the rage I have inside. The disease I have is so fucking raw. She's able to uncover it. When she's standing there and I'm at the liquor store and I have the fucking bottle in my hand, and she has her hand on it, I'm like, get your hands off me.

How are you feeling about abstinence now?

So I'm home now. I'm waiting on the school bus for the kid. What ran through my mind was, 'Oh, my God, the liquor store to the left is five minutes away and the liquor store to the right is five minutes away.' So the first day I got out after six weeks I thought of vodka and alcohol. And I'm saying to myself that I've been away for a month, and when I was there I didn't think about alcohol once.

That's one of the limitations of rehab, that you have to get out.

Well, yeah, it's actually like getting out of prison. And then I couldn't believe it because that's people, places, and things. Because I used to think, 'Oh My God, the bus is coming. I can get to the liquor store after the bus gets here.'

Could AA overcome this? Although the meetings helped him stay on course, it took much effort in counseling with him and his wife to establish some equanimity in the home, and in tactfully helping her understand that Carl's program had to be his own; she had to pull back. In time, Carl reconciled himself as best he could to the limitations he lived with, and began to accommodate himself to sobriety. He would discuss the guilt he felt over the compromise he had brought upon his wife and his child, but he always did feel some pressure to drink.

TRYING BUT FAILING

AA stalwarts have always said that alcoholism is a fatal disease. And so it can be, despite the best efforts of the afflicted person to make use of the fellowship, and even with all the professional help one can get. This was true for Jessica, a talented artist, who diligently went to meetings and persisted in psychotherapy, but would repeatedly relapse nonetheless.

She was the daughter of a prominent and overbearing playwright who favored her over her brothers to the point of having her sleep in his bed, albeit without sexual contact, until she was thirteen. Ultimately, she rebelled against her father during her adolescence and young adulthood, and had affairs with some of the litterati in his social circle. Over the course of her adult years, she was never able to establish a long-lasting stable relationship with a mate.

Jessica drank alone at home, and very heavily, often awakening with no recollection of when she had lapsed into a drunk stupor. She could achieve periods of abstinence, but would inevitably fall back into a damaging relapse, sometimes leaving her inaccessible for a day or two. All this, despite her earnest attempts to deal diligently with her problem. She clearly tried hard to make the fellowship work for her, even attending AA retreats on occasion, but she remained ambivalent about the fellowship, unable to dispel a feeling of it being intrusive and, similar to her Dad, overbearing. She also was never able to switch from a sponsor who was demanding a more devout commitment to AA prayer than she felt she could sustain. In a way, she saw me as a kindly and supportive figure, splitting her feelings and identifying AA somehow as the oppressor. In actuality, people in her home group were most supportive of her, even moving the meeting to her apartment one time when she had fallen and broken her leg while drunk.

Jessica was able to sustain a highly compromised existence. Her paintings were sought after and they sold well through her agent. An inheritance from her father assured that she had the financial support she needed during periods when her drinking left her unproductive. But her well-being was never assured during the three years I saw her in therapy. Despite two attempts at rehab, each successful for a time, her relapses both times left her more physically compromised, and her life in greater disarray. If I was away for a week on business, she would drink herself into a stuporous state, and on two occasions I had the police (and me as well) come to her apartment to retrieve her when she was inaccessible. In our sessions, I tried as best I could to deal with her inclination to see my being away as potential vacations from abstinence.

So, sadly, she eventually did drink to a level of alcohol poisoning, having consumed more than her body could sustain. The last time that I called the police to her door, while anticipating my arrival as well, she was no longer alive. In the end, she tragically proved the lethal potential of her disease.

Could more have been done? I had spoken with colleagues seeking opinions on what might be done to help her more effectively. In fact, when I suggested at one point that she might do well to see a different therapist, she refused to do so. Would some other course of treatment have done better at saving her life? Should I have pressed her more pointedly to get a more appropriate sponsor? One cannot help but wonder if alternatives might have been pursued. Most of us who have treated addiction for years have had to confront questions like these.

In AA's most recent triennial survey, 48% of those responding had been sober for six or more years. How long do people really need to continue going to meetings? Some, as we have seen in previous chapters, continue in an open-ended way. Typically, they intuitively "know" that relapse would befall them if they stopped attending. I suspect that they are right. If this works for them, and they feel they need it, who would rightly ask them to stop? But there is more than one way to maintain a lifelong commitment. One man went to daily meetings for his first five years, but later tapered off, and now provides service for the fellowship. He attends meetings only two or three times a month, goes to AA retreats on occasion, and is an officer in his local intergroup. He made this observation about open-ended attendance:

> The majority of people stop going or severely cut back after a period, but can maintain their sobriety anyway. Some people have trouble bringing the fundamentals of recovery into the rest of their lives, or find the AA meetings comforting, or act on the side of safety.

"Acting on the side of safety:" Why do these daily attenders need to go so frequently for so long? We will never know for sure; they have made their own judgments as best they can.

It is interesting to consider two other options in the context of long-term sobriety: championing recovery in the public forum, or no longer going to meetings but remaining abstinent. William Cope Moyers, who directs Hazelden's Center for Public Advocacy, has pursued the first of these options, and he described the second in someone whom he knew.

Moyers is a cogent and inspiring speaker, with a striking story of his own, which he tells in his book, *Broken*.[25] In his early twenties he had to be admitted to Hazelden rehab, but he relapsed onto multiple drugs some two years later. After a second rehab admission, he married, had two kids, and pursued a promising career in journalism. One day, though, he impulsively bought some crack cocaine and lapsed into addiction again. This time, he ended up in a crack house, and, as he wrote, "hadn't shaved, showered, or eaten for four days." His parents refused to give up on him, and had him extracted from the crack house by two off-duty police, after which they had him brought to a third episode of rehab. This time his recovery stuck, and now, twenty years of sobriety later, he is a national leader for improved addiction treatment, giving talks countrywide and testifying before Congress to advance that cause.

Although still a dedicated AA member, he realizes that Twelve Step recovery cannot be bound by rigid adherence to a narrowly defined path. He suggested that dropping out of regular attendance after years of sobriety can be an option for some members, as he described to me—

> ... a woman who got sober at 22, and she's been sober for over thirty years now. She was a mainstay in my home group, was full of wisdom, and had a lot of joy and a lot of real world experience. Two years ago she stopped coming, and she hasn't been back. And I called her not too long ago, and she said, "I'm tired of the same old thing. I have no desire to take a drink; I have no desire to go back to the old days in my behavior. I've kind of moved on, and I respect AA and I try to live by those principles. She said that she was tired of hearing people talking about the same old thing, and I can understand that. A lot of old-timers in AA will say that when you start to think like that and start talking that way you are going to relapse. I disagree.

He told me:

> If AA wants to be relevant to the largest number of addicts and alcoholics in this country, it will need, if not to embrace, then to understand the changing dynamics of addiction treatment and recovery. It needs to be able to see the realities of the intersection between science, research, spirituality, and history. Otherwise, it will continue to be a relevant program, but just be relevant to a smaller number of people.

On this count, Moyers endorses Hazelden's introduction of monthly injections of the opiate blocker depot naltrexone (Vivitrol) and, alternatively, daily opioid maintenance (Suboxone) for some of the Center's painkiller- and heroin-addicted patients. Hazelden is in many ways the Mecca for Twelve-Step-based recovery, and this new approach has been developed in the context of an AA-based treatment system, and combined with AA participation. What Moyers says is quite telling in relation to how Twelve Step-based rehabs are evolving, and may well operate in the future.

METHADONE ANONYMOUS

Here is one potential modification. At New York University and Bellevue Hospital, we wanted to engage the strength of the Twelve Step spiritually based recovery for our patients on methadone maintenance. Methadone patients are typically not accepted in AA meetings; many members think they are on no more than another addictive drug. I had heard that there were some Twelve Step groups operating for patients enrolled in some of the city's methadone clinics, so we surveyed members of these groups and evaluated the nature of their membership. Their responses indicated that they rated the Twelve Step components as more helpful to their recovery than the components of the methadone programs.[26]

We then set up a protocol for "Methadone Anonymous," a Twelve-Step-based program in our methadone clinic, coordinated by a counselor who was himself in Twelve Step recovery. We received support from the National Institute of Drug Abuse to assess it. Two aspects of the program were quite telling.[27] Those patients who became engaged developed a zeal for recovery, for improved involvement in the community, and for seeking employment. They stood in contrast to most of the clinic patients, who were typically alienated from the clinic's mission of pursuing re-entry into community life, and who viewed the program pretty much as a source for the dependency-producing agent (methadone) we were dispensing.

Although the program's external government support was terminated after two years, and there was no pressure from the clinic administration for it to be continued, it had staying power. Even now, fifteen years later, it continues to operate with enthusiastic participation of members who attend its meetings. The AA ethos can survive and flourish under surprisingly diverse circumstances.

WHAT IS RECOVERY?

"I'm in recovery," is how many AA members describe how they are doing once they have stopped drinking or using drugs for a long time. What they mean to say is that they have not already "recovered" from a disease, because they view addiction as a lifelong vulnerability. In fact, members acknowledge this limitation even if they have already found a satisfactory and stable adaptation in their sober state. The fellowship defines itself in the Big Book as a way of developing a "new way of living" with its prescribed spiritual course; it does not say that the new way of living means that one is cured.

But in practical terms, people have to know whether a job applicant who needed treatment for drinking or drugs will be reliable as a potential employee. Even future spouses may want to consider how much they can rely on someone who says that they have been to rehab, that they are going to AA meetings, or that they do not drink because they "used to have a problem with alcohol."

Tom McClellan, a leader in studying the nature of addiction and the effectiveness of its treatment, realized that people in the government who plan for health care, as well as employers and insurers, use the term recovery at times, but with no consensus on just what it means. He decided to lend some definition to it by convening a group of experts to see whether they could come up with a way of defining it. It was a diverse group, some members from academic research, others from the treatment field, and also a representative from the Betty Ford rehab center, where the meeting was held. Members ranged from people who did not treat addicted people to addicted people who were "in recovery." As one of the panel members, I was impressed by the diversity and good sense represented there.

We came up with what seemed like a useful consensus.[28] First, a person had to be "sober," that is, refraining from alcohol and other nonprescribed drugs. The panel agreed that *prescribed* medications like methadone or naltrexone, taken voluntarily, did not remove a person from under the umbrella definition of recovery. This was important because it acknowledged the legitimacy of opioid maintenance and of blocking agents that many members in community-based Twelve Step groups were reluctant to accept. Second, people had to be in "personal health," broadly meaning an improved quality of physical and psychological well-being. Finally, they had to be good "citizens," living with respect for those around them. If the recovering person had achieved this overall status for a year, then using the terminology of the American Psychiatric Association (DSM-IV), they were in "sustained remission." After five years, they are defined as in "stable remission."

This initiative could be valuable to people in recovery, because it relieved them of living under the shadow of the limitations imputed to a lifelong illness by acknowledging that there can be a state where their recovery is validated by what they had achieved. It did not have an explicit specific basis in hard research, but frankly, neither do the health-related evaluations we have for many other ailments. We speak of five-year survival rates for cancers, but many malignancies can return years later; stents are used to keep blocked arteries working well, but cardiac problems can return nonetheless; depression, successfully treated one time, can recur years later. Relieving the body and mind of their ailments is not as definitive as one would hope. Nonetheless, at some point, people do have to accord themselves, and be accorded, some sense that their well-being is reasonably stabilized and acceptable.

Lee Ann Kaskutas, a member of the panel, decided to poll people who designated themselves as "in recovery," to see how they defined this for themselves. One might surmise that their definition of their own status, also not subjected to empirical testing, is as legitimate as that of the experts. She and her colleagues polled over 9,000 people who said they were "in recovery." These people had been solicited through e-mail, ads in the media, and recovery-oriented organizations—but not through AA itself, because it does not collaborate with researchers.[29] They found that most of the people responding viewed recovery pretty much the same way that the expert panel did, as abstinence-based, but importantly, not all indicated that full abstinence was required. Some drinking, even some use of drugs, was acceptable to 9% of the alcoholic respondents. They had been just as likely to meet the psychiatric criteria for alcohol dependence when they were actively addicted as the rest.

CHAPTER 13

Other Options

Since the 1930s, the usual course of an AA encounter has gone as follows: Someone has a problem with alcohol. His doctor, or maybe his irate spouse, tells him to go to AA. Maybe he himself decides to go. He goes to some meetings; perhaps he stays on; he may later get a sponsor and work the Steps. This is what we have reviewed here so far, but there obviously are other possibilities for pursuing a course toward recovery from alcoholism. We will now consider some of these alternatives. Some are compatible with AA membership, and others are not. Here are some of the options we will consider.

At most AA meetings, members cannot really talk openly about drugs other than alcohol. Thus, Narcotics Anonymous (NA) was developed by heroin addicts in the 1940s to offer the benefits of the Twelve Step format for people addicted to drugs other than alcohol. Nowadays, addicts of any and all drugs, from heroin and cocaine to newer pharmaceuticals like pain-killers, are welcomed in NA. Their meetings differ very little or not at all from the AA format.

There are also fellowship options that reflect the transition that has occurred since the culture of the 1930s, when Protestant revivalism had a major influence on Bill W and Dr. Bob. These other programs relieve their members of having to turn their "will and lives" over to a higher power. They vary from an agnostic adaptation of AA, to fellowships that do not use the Twelve Steps for promoting abstinence, to one that helps people moderate their drinking rather than stop completely. Some of these alternative fellowships draw on the example of the mutual support that AA offers, but promote the option of modifying its basic tenets.

We will also consider some of the ways doctors and other professionals on their own help alcoholic patients get free of addiction. They may draw primarily on a patient's family and close friends to support a person's abstinence, and they also can use medications or a structured talk therapy. These approaches can be applied along with AA, or without it. They reflect how physicians and psychologists have begun to think about ways they can apply their professional techniques to a problem that in the past they had either avoided or had been left at a loss as to how to treat. They draw on developments in psychotherapy and pharmacology that emerged long after Bill W and Bob found that they had only each other to rely on.

NARCOTICS ANONYMOUS

For a person whose primary problem is drugs other than alcohol, this fellowship is a readily accessible option, with some 50,000 groups world-wide.[1] In our survey of NA members, we found that the most common drug problem reported was cocaine, followed by heroin. However, even alcohol was reported as a primary drug problem for 9% of the members.[2] Like AA, NA employs the Twelve Step format, and its meetings are generally conducted in a similar way. In fact, NA emerged out of drug-addicted people's attempts to adapt the AA principles to their problems.

The program's history can be traced back to its origins on the federal Lexington, Kentucky narcotics farm, as is described in its own literature[3] and in a scholarly study by William White.[4] (White is an astute historian of the many attempts to treat addiction, from Benjamin Rush, a doctor who was a signatory to the Declaration of Independence, up to the present.)

In the 1930s, heroin addicts could go to a federal facility in Lexington in an attempt to divorce themselves from their compulsive drug-seeking; most were sent there under pressure from the courts. Among other things, the facility served as the site for some of the key medical studies that were designed to understand how drugs, opiates in particular, affected the physiology of people addicted to them. The residents at Lexington, though, were not without initiative of their own to address their addiction, and some thought that adopting AA's Twelve Steps to their problem represented a reasonable option. Ultimately, when discharged from Lexington, some of the addicts drew together in groups that later coalesced into an organized network. Some initially called themselves Addicts Anonymous, but not wanting to confuse their name with the acronym of AA, they inserted "Narcotics" into their name. Their Steps were virtually the same as AA's, but they substituted "we were powerless over our addiction" for "powerless over alcohol."

They corresponded with AA's headquarters to solicit use of its literature, but the stigma attached to heroin addiction was much greater than that of alcoholism. Because of this, members of either group seeking recovery at that time were unlikely to be formally associated with one another. Heroin addicts were seen more as criminally bound to their drug of choice and members of an underclass, unlike the AA members, who were quite happy to avoid association with the heroin addicts. In the end, Bill W wrote in the AA *Grapevine* magazine[5] that a line had to be drawn that would limit AA to including only alcohol addicts. But this is now often observed in the breach.

NA now has people under its worldwide umbrella who are addicted to a variety of drugs of abuse and who originate from a wide array of social class backgrounds and subcultures. The stigma for some was hard to shake off, as illustrated by the fact that the Narcotics Anonymous Handbook, one early attempt at preparing an equivalent of AA's Big Book, was developed by prison inmates in California rather than by civilians in the community. The book's current counterpart, titled *Narcotics Anonymous,* of which the sixth edition[6] is now in print, is organized like the AA Big Book in that the first half deals with general issues, and the second half deals with experiences of some exemplary members.

Many American members of NA come from disadvantaged backgrounds while others do not. One Vietnam army veteran in NA recovery, still unemployed, described his attempt to escape from alienation:

> My household was very bad. We were poor and I got beaten as a kid. My father carried a gun, and so did I after a while. I started drinking beer when I was eight and joined a street gang. Then I joined the Army to get away, but brought drugs with me. While I was in combat, in the service, I got hooked on heroin, alcohol, and everything else. I got high and crashed one of the vehicles because I was out partying. They sent me to Phoenix House [a therapeutic community]. Being a Vietnam vet was really hard because everyone was negative about Vietnam, and I felt it through and through. Even though the program gives you the Twelve Steps, you have to talk about how you feel. . . . I could talk about my Vietnam experience with my sponsor, the way I couldn't with anyone outside the rooms. I have a safe place, and put myself together straight.

In contrast, some members of NA come from mainstream middle-class backgrounds, but they, too, ultimately succumbed to the ravages of uncontrolled drug use:

> I grew up in a small town in New England in an intact family; no alcohol or drug abuse by my parents. I graduated high school with honors; captain of the cheerleader squad, went to nursing school. . . .

My husband Ben was a Vietnam veteran, and he was exposed to heroin over there. One day I walked into the house. I was like, "What are you guys doing?" He said, "Well, it's my birthday and we're going to do a little heroin." I said, "Heroin?" I watched them, and then they asked if I wanted to try a little. I felt like what a lot of people in recovery will say, I felt whole. I felt like, wow, I have been searching for you my whole life. . . .

I had to start stealing checks and forging the signatures. I was a really good forger. . . . I was also a booster, stealing stuff like Lenox china from stores and turning around and walking back later and returning it for cash. . . . Being that I had gone to finishing school for six months, I could dress for the part and act the part, so that I would be above suspicion . . .

In jail, I detoxed cold turkey in solitary confinement for about two weeks, hallucinated, ran a fever, visual and auditory hallucinations, no food, couldn't eat, couldn't talk. After release, I got a job in a corporate medical department and stole a prescription pad, and put on a nursing uniform to pick up prescriptions. I went on and off methadone, and got arrested again. The judge gave me the choice of going to NA or going back to prison, so I decided I would go to NA until I was done with parole, and along the way, I got to enjoy living life. Needless to say, I have had therapy four times . . . I've been sober for twelve years. I must say, life in NA is going well for me now.

One of the presidents of the American Society of Addiction Medicine was in Twelve Step recovery and was committed to promoting cooperation between doctors and AA. He introduced me to representatives of the NA central office at one conference, and vouched for me as someone who could understand their program. Unlike AA, with its Traditions, NA's World Service Office can cooperate with a researcher if they choose to do so. I asked if NA would let me carry out an assessment of the background of their members and the nature of their experience in the fellowship. Given the studies I had done on addiction recovery, the NA hierarchy agreed to help with this, and sent a survey of ours to NA groups in four different states. When we analyzed our findings,[7] we found that spiritual awakening in long-term NA members and the nature of their stable sobriety was very much like that of the AA members we had studied.

Because NA's central office had been cooperative in helping set up this initial study, I asked whether they could arrange a focus group with NA members so that my research group and I could get a firsthand sense of how these members would describe their experience in the program. As it happened, seven of the nine NA people who participated had been in the military during the Vietnam era. For some, their substance abuse had led to a dishonorable discharge. Others fell into addiction, even homelessness, after separating from the service. All had described an experience of alienation on returning to civilian life, often with symptoms of post-traumatic stress disorder (PTSD). They left a compelling impression of how the fellowship could respond to this particularly alienated group of people: While in NA, they became part of a lineage that could transmit their experience of recovery from one generation of veterans to the next. As one of them said,

> When I came back, I hated my country. I couldn't talk about the Vietnam experience, and kept a lot of things inside, but I could talk to my sponsor about things I was going through because he was in the military. The program has taught me to just give back, to get myself back to some kind of normality; I couldn't have done it without God. . . . The guys coming from Iraq get the benefit of us Vietnam vets and we help them come home and get back into society.

I discussed the experiences that these veterans reported with my liaison from the NA central office, and she agreed that it would be important to document this for the members with service-related symptoms, given that NA was generally an underutilized resource within the VA medical system.

The NA office was able to access sixteen groups in five different states that had a representation of veterans. Over two thirds of the veterans had originally needed hospitalization for alcohol or drug problems, and over two thirds also reported symptoms that related to PTSD. They documented the same experience of renewal in the fellowship that our focus group members had described.[8]

PTSD and drug abuse were highly publicized problems for veterans returning from the wars in the Middle East, and it seemed that increasing access to NA as a resource for dealing with this would be quite valuable. This is particularly the case because the techniques[9] being developed and used for this issue inevitably take more professional staffing than can be fully provided.

I spoke with some key members I knew in the VA psychiatry system, and they were quite interested in our findings. We discussed the value of accessing information on how many of the vets they were treating were actually attending Twelve Step meetings. Despite the orientation of the VA toward computerization for better retrieval of patient information, it became clear that no such information was available; nor for that matter, was long-term follow-up information on their addicted patients' outcomes systematically recorded. Deficits in outcome information are most unfortunate, because this leaves the system without access to findings that would be valuable in making clinical decisions. (We have the same lack of long-term outcome information in the civilian realm.)

The scope of NA's international reach is also impressive, and it illustrates the fellowship's particular importance in the many countries where drug problems are more common than alcohol ones. The situation in Iran is an interesting example of this. Heroin addiction is highly pervasive there, and NA has a big footprint in that country. I was quite taken by the fact the NA's central office tabulations showed that there were 17,000 NA groups in Iran, second only to the United States in number, where there are 26,000.

I was introduced to NA's coordinator for Iran at an international conference and asked him about how the fellowship operated in Iran, hoping to get an idea of why it has so much of a presence there. He explained that in Iran, members form supportive networks among themselves in addition to their regular meetings. Sponsors routinely get together with their sponsees as a group to see how they can help one another outside of the regular meetings and to see if family members could be helped. He explained that this reflected the closely knit family and social ties that are in place for providing mutual help, a very important part of traditional Iranian culture.

This was instructive in understanding how in a country like the United States, where people are increasingly alienated from ties with friends and neighbors, Twelve Step mutual support is less intensive outside meetings than in a country with more active and persistent ties among friends and families. Needless to say, the fellowship's population there also illustrates the adaptability of NA to a non-Christian setting, where one's understanding of a higher power can be seen as compatible with the people's commitment to the deity they worship.

AA WITHOUT "GOD"

Randy, a successful corporate consultant, had progressed over time from social drinking to bingeing. He sustained a career in the firm he had founded largely because of his specialization in a particular area of marketing for which he had unique expertise. He came to realize, though, that his drinking habit was heading the wrong way, particularly in his family life. This became all too clear after he showed up at home around 2 AM several times after "innocently" stopping off at a bar for a few drinks on the way home from work. It was all the more compelling that he remembered little of what had happened during those missing hours.

Randy had managed to stop drinking a few times for several days, but he would always fall back into it. When he came for consultation, he was several days sober this time as well, but said he knew he could not sustain it on his own. He saw coming for help as a sensible decision, an extension of the good judgment he applied in his business ventures.

It is hard to know what role AA will play in a person's recovery after she or he is encouraged to attend several meetings. Not all will continue to attend consistently. Many will not go so far as to get a sponsor. I have certainly found, though, that for most of those who attend some meetings when they are at a stage like Randy's, it can help them get clear on the need to adopt a positive outlook on the value of abstinence. So I asked Randy to go to two or three meetings before we met the next week, not being sure how he would experience them, even after my giving him an explanation of what he might expect.

When Randy returned a week later, he had gone to two meetings and had not drunk in the interim. He said he had found the meetings interesting, and might have been open to attending further, but was turned off by all that talk about "the little guy up in the sky." He saw himself as agnostic, even an atheist, and because of this, he was ambivalent about going back.

We have little information on how many people across the country attend AA after referral by professionals, but clearly, exposure to the fellowship is quite common among alcoholics getting help for their drinking. One analysis of data from a large federal survey is informative in this regard.[10] Of people who experienced the onset of alcohol dependence at some point during the previous year, 26% of those surveyed indicated that they had received some type of help. Two thirds of that group reported that they had participated in both treatment and Twelve Step groups, more than had gone to treatment only or only to the fellowships. We have no findings from this survey on how many continued with either option. Neither do we know how many balk, upon their first encounters with AA, at the role ascribed to a higher power. Some certainly are uncomfortable with the issue. Randy fell into this latter group of attendees in that he combined treatment and AA, but he was uncomfortable with the issue of "God, as we understood Him."

What were some options for Randy, the agnostic? The AA Agnostica[11] website has become a resource for people in Twelve Step recovery who value the support and the fidelity that the fellowship provides its members, but are not prepared to accept its commitment to a God, even if it is "*as we understood Him*." The website includes a citation from Bill's writing in the book, *Alcoholics Anonymous Comes of Age*[12]: "We must remember that AA's steps are suggestions only. A belief in them is not at all a requirement for membership among us." The Agnostica website then lists a number of modified versions of the Steps, for example, "We came to believe and accept that we needed strengths beyond our awareness and resources" rather than "a Power greater than ourselves." The website also provides information on the fellowship's growing number of meetings in the United States, overseas, and online. In Randy's case, AA Agnostica offered thirteen meetings in New York City.

The issue of agnosticism in AA is not a new one. As early as 1938, when one of two AA groups of the nascent fellowship was located in New York under the leadership of Bill W, and the other in Akron, where Dr. Bob lived, the issue was brought up by Jim Burwell in New York who had just joined the fellowship. As a self-proclaimed atheist he objected to God-related terminology in the Steps, and pressed Bill W to offer an adaptation that would temper the pressure to proclaim fidelity to a deity. Bill modified the Steps accordingly by adding the phrase "as we understood Him," and reduced the mentions of God in the Steps from six to four. He also altered the Seventh Step—"Humbly asked him to remove our shortcomings"—by removing the phrase "on our knees." The Big Book also got a whole chapter, "We Agnostics." If one reads the chapter, though, one sees that it presumes that the nonbeliever will in time come around to accept God in some fashion. It ends with the tale of a man who "thought he was an atheist." In his misery in the hospital he tumbles out of bed and ultimately finds himself "in conscious companionship with his Creator."

A key for validating the non-theistic AA groups also can be seen in the Twelve Traditions, AA's governing philosophy, which states that "the only requirement for AA membership is a desire to stop drinking," with no mention of having to accept a Higher Power in one's life. Conflicts have arisen, though, on the issue of which AA groups are listed by AA intergroups in their local brochures and on the Internet. Such a listing effectively gives a group validation as a legitimate component of the AA flock. In some areas, agnostic groups were "de-listed," and in other areas, the differences in outlook have been overlooked.

Ernie Kurtz wrote the most thorough history of AA, from its inception to its recent years.[13] He had been a doctoral candidate in the history of religion in America at Harvard in the late 1970s, and became aware of AA while doing some marriage counseling, as he had a master's degree in psychology as well. The director of the Hazelden rehab center, whom Kurtz encountered at one point during his studies, told him about the AA archives at the fellowship's central office in New York. Kurtz followed up on this lead, and, as he told me, found a "graduate student's dream, the unviewed documents of a major American movement."

Both Kurtz and Bill White, a historian of addiction treatment, spoke of the importance they attributed to AA Agnostica and the liberalization movement it represented in terms of the evolution of AA. They also jointly wrote an introduction to the book, *Don't Tell,* [14] which includes a compilation of personal stories from the AA Agnostica website.

AA is a fellowship where fidelity and respect for those who commit themselves to leadership is very important. Although Kurtz was not a member, his history of AA[15] gave him a special place among its members, and his acceptance of the agnostic group is important. *A History of Agnostic Groups in AA*[16] is available as an e-book, and Kurtz wrote its author warmly saying that, "The fellowship owes you a debt of gratitude, though it may take time for them to realize it." This quote is featured prominently on the AA Agnostica website.

Kurtz and White both spoke with me about a tension in AA, as some members whom they referred to as "fundamentalists" or "Christianizers" have gone the opposite way of liberalization, introducing the Lord's Prayer in meetings and insisting on a particular kind of spiritual awakening. In my discussions with members from Middle America, as opposed to the two coasts, many quite clearly saw AA's Higher Power as essentially the same as the Christian deity worshiped in the churches in which they grew up.

On the other hand, some members have adopted a Buddhist outlook on the Steps. Unlike the Biblical prophets, Buddha is not seen as speaking for a supernatural creator. Instead, he is understood to be an enlightened teacher who can lead people to a "right way of living," a spiritually oriented course to relieve the suffering that comes from worldly and material desire. This is a message that also can refer to relief of the craving for alcohol, and can be combined with the Buddhist practice of meditation, two elements that are compatible with AA's philosophy.

The AA General Service Conference has tried to define the boundaries of the spirituality it espouses, and its policies were recently spelled out in one of its leaflets under the heading, "Many Paths to Spirituality." The following makes clear how a Buddhist orientation, even perhaps an agnostic one, could be acceptable within the fellowship:

> Many of us came to rely on a "Higher Power," whether it was the collective power of A.A., the A.A. group itself, or some other entity, concept or being that helped us to stay sober. . . . Many of us come from different belief systems and cultures, yet there has always been plenty of latitude in A.A. for members to practice whatever belief works best for them.[17]

The compatibility of the Twelve Steps with Buddhist philosophy is illustrated in some recent books. One[18] describes the conflict experienced by a woman who came to espouse a Buddhist approach. She had trouble accepting the concept of God even "as we understood Him," and instead wrote that she saw her commitment to God to be embodied in the fellowship's members. For her, GOD meant a "Group Of Drunks." She wrote that the prayer and meditation of the Eleventh Step can be seen in seeking mindfulness as it is defined these days. Experiencing mindfulness is important in Buddhism. She described it as a way of focusing on one's thoughts and feelings of the moment, and thereby providing relief from preoccupation with one's worldly self. This way, Buddhist meditation can fit in comfortably with what one is seeking through the Steps. If more evidence for the acceptability of this outlook were needed, it is provided by Hazelden, the best known of the rehab centers. The website of its publishing arm offers a book called *Mindfulness and the Twelve Steps*.[19] Its author, with Zen training, has carried out related retreats at the Hazelden's Renewal Center on its main campus in Minnesota.

Buddhism also can serve as a path to follow on the way *out* of the fellowship, and AA Agnostica offers an option that could lead that way. On its website, in "A Buddhist's Views on AA," one can read that the fellowship:

> . . . routinely risks becoming quasi-religious, institutionalized, and bent upon its own survival at the expense of actually helping people recover. . . . In a sense, AA has acquired an ego and now finds itself in the difficult struggle to sustain relevance in a Universe that no longer fully subscribes to its world view . . . to elevate the literature to sacred-text status that makes even the most benign constructive criticism unacceptable.

The AA Agnostica website offers the Buddhist, non-theistic Twelve Steps: "came to believe that a power other than the self [is] ready to work at transforming ourselves," replaces to "have God remove all these defects of character." A path like this out the fellowship is fully expressed in one book[20] by an author who left AA and stayed sober. She writes that she can quote the Big Book "with the best of them,"[21] but has moved on to reading the classic Tibetan Buddhist texts. She strives to improve contact with her own "center of awareness," instead of improving her "conscious contact with God."

AA as a popular movement has been around for over seventy-five years and has survived remarkably well, much of it due to the foresight of Bill W in framing its Twelve Traditions. He included in them, "Our common welfare should come first; personal recovery depends on AA unity." But the fellowship did emerge from the experience of its two cofounders in the Oxford Group, whose members avowed a strongly felt system of Christian beliefs. The Oxford Group was not, however, a religion, nor was it a part of any religious domination. Many AA members came to be comfortable, or at least accepting, of its somewhat softened view of a deity. As one person many years sober in the program said to me, "It doesn't matter who your Higher Power is, as long as it's not you."

ABSTINENCE WITHOUT THE TWELVE STEPS

The middle third of the twentieth century was a period when a wide variety of views were emerging on how to address problems related to alcoholism. Prohibition was coming to an end, and it was thought that it was better to let liquor flow to drinkers, even alcoholics, who had been in some measure of hiding; the alternative would have meant continuing to support burgeoning crime syndicates. Meanwhile, esteemed psychiatrists of the day were beginning to realize that alcoholics were not responsive to their lauded instrument, the psychoanalytic technique. Medical scientists in the federal addiction farm in Lexington, Kentucky were developing biologic approaches to understanding how addiction works. And of course, Bill W and Dr Bob were struggling to save each other's souls.

Another approach was also emerging. The psychologist Albert Ellis, who practiced on his own outside an academic setting, was conceiving of a technique called Rational Emotive Therapy.[22] It was premised on the idea that although adverse experiences can produce distress, the nature of their impact depends on how much a person believes in what they mean. If such events lead him or her to see guilt and failure in everyday events, it is not surprising that these adverse experiences will leave the person depressed.

Ellis, however, thought that rationality could be introduced into the way depressed people interpret events, thereby helping them to dispel their pessimistic connotations and relieving them of their suffering. It actually worked rather well, and the approach ultimately was elaborated and researched as cognitive behavioral therapy by Aaron Beck, an academic psychiatrist.[23]

A number of abstinence-oriented programs based on this approach, which present an alternative to AA, have arisen in recent years. The most obvious commonality among them is that they do not use the Twelve Steps and they do not rely on commitment to a higher power. Some, but not all, recognize the importance of stopping the use of alcohol and other drugs. These approaches are in line with a disposition toward secularism, which has gained more of a voice in the public domain since the mid-1930s. I would like to illustrate this approach with Rational Recovery, which ceased to operate when its leader decided to reorganize it along for-profit lines, and a successor program, SMART Recovery, which has achieved a good measure of success.

By the mid-1960s, Jack Trimpey, a recovering alcoholic social worker living in California, had achieved sobriety while attending AA, but was balking at the program's God-centered focus. He developed a format for Rational Recovery groups, drawing on Albert Ellis's cognitively based model. Trimpey maintained that a person could gain control over his drinking by disregarding the presumption of powerlessness put forward by AA, and not having to deal with a deity or the presumption of spiritual deficits.

Trimpey personified the compulsive thoughts that drive the alcoholic to drink as "The Beast." He found that people in a supportive group setting could apply an approach to separating themselves from that instinct-like, pressing feeling, and strengthen their will to not drink. The idea here was for the person to come to realize that, "I don't want to drink; the Beast wants me to, and I can put it off." As if to dismiss and mock AA's format, Trimpey wrote a book spelling out his approach and titled it "The Small Book."[24] In his hands, Rational Recovery had considerable appeal for many people who shared his aversion to Higher Power issues, and many were no doubt relieved that the ninety-minute meetings only took place on a weekly basis, rather than the more frequent occurrences that AA had prescribed.

Trimpey and I met, and he was interested in my offer of having his program studied to document its presumed success. Along with colleagues, I was able to poll members in sixty-three of his ongoing groups. Of those who had joined three months or more before, 73% had been abstinent in the previous month, and had attended an average of one meeting a week. This was most notable. Also notable was that those members who had been abstinent for at least three months had at one point in the past attended an average of twenty AA meetings in a month. It looked like the stability of many Rational Recovery participants was based in good part on their previous experience in AA, even though they had become disenchanted with the "God talk" there.

Unlike Rational Recovery, Bill W's fellowship owed some of its success to the fact that it never got embedded in a for-profit residential or hospital-based setting. This may be due as much to the fact that Bill could not raise the funds early on to initiate that course as to his relative wisdom. At a time when rehabs were emerging a quarter century later, Jack Trimpey saw things otherwise. Five years after we did our research, he announced that group meetings were in his judgment unproductive, and that his groups were coming to an end. This coincided with his opening a for-profit residential setting with stays between one and three months. The program's brochure touted that its location in the foothills of the Sierra Nevada Mountains meant that it was only an hour away from Lake Tahoe, a location that was famous for "skiing, show business, and casinos." So much for the incentive to mix the profit motive with a rehab setting.

SMART Recovery is a nonprofit, abstinence-oriented organization that emerged as Rational Recovery was changing its course. This new nonprofit program also disavows the spiritual orientation of AA, and emphasizes a cognitive approach like the rational emotive and cognitive behavioral therapies. It views alcohol dependence from the perspective of a bad and compelling habit, rather than a disease, as such. Meetings are run by facilitators, preferably professionals, which stands in contrast to AA where group leadership is elected for limited periods among the recovering alcoholics who belong to the group. One recent survey[25] sheds some light on the program. Alcohol is the most common drug of abuse and one third of respondents reported using AA as well as SMART Recovery. An online option using the SMART Recovery format is available, and 40% who responded say they relied on this more than on face-to-face meetings. On the positive side, SMART Recovery has the appeal of being open to research-based treatment approaches. However, it lacks the aspect of active mutual support provided by AA with its personalized help from other members and access to a supportive sponsor. AA also offers meetings at almost any time in any neighborhood in many cities, a resource that SMART Recovery does not have.

AA's social aspect underlies its ability to recruit new members. For this reason, the emergence of AA Agnostica provides an interesting contrast to SMART Recovery. On the plus side, the agnostic groups offer the easy access to support that their parent fellowship, AA, has. On the other hand, they are more demanding in terms of time and commitment than the cognitively oriented alternative. Research that can give a reliable picture of the relative effectiveness of the two approaches, and follow-up what happens to people who engage in these two respective options over time, remains to be conducted. In any case, even using their own figures, AA has about 2,000 times as many weekly meetings as SMART Recovery to choose from, yet SMART Recovery has continued to expand rapidly since its inception in 1992. There is room for both.

MODERATION MANAGEMENT

In 1994, two years after SMART Recovery was founded, a woman named Audrey Kishline started a group program for people with alcohol problems, but this one was for people who wanted to cut back on their drinking rather than stop entirely. Her own experience illustrates the quandary of where to draw the line between people who can successfully moderate and those who cannot deal with their drinking problem without full abstinence.

Six years after founding the program, Kishline apparently realized that for her at least, limited drinking was not working. She posted a message for the program's members that she supported the program for those who could moderate successfully, but that she herself had to stop drinking, and was going to AA. Not long thereafter, as if to tragically demonstrate the risks associated with unabated alcoholism, she drove drunk the wrong way down a highway, hit another car, and killed the driver and his 12-year-old daughter. For this she went to prison.[26]

Clearly, though, not all people who drink in a problematic way have the kind of alcohol problem for which abstinence is the only option. Many can and do cut back with or without a program's support. As we discussed in the chapter addressing whether alcoholism is a disease, some people meet the criteria that the federal government considers to define heavy drinkers, but not all would necessarily be considered alcoholic. Here is how much the government's institute for alcoholism thinks you should drink to qualify as a heavy drinker: for men, more than four drinks on any day, or more than fourteen in a week; for women the figures are three drinks a day and seven in a week.[27] Federal figures also point out that although 25% of adults qualify as binge drinkers, only 7% can be defined as having what they call an "alcohol use disorder."[28]

Moderation Management (MM) did continue on after its founder's auto accident, and its website points out that for many people, early intervention can prevent a decline into alcoholic-level drinking, a syndrome that is much harder to treat. It posits that one may be suitable for membership if one can check off items like: you have interests and other ways to relax besides drinking, you never drink secretly, and you usually do not drink for more than an hour or two on a particular occasion.[29] MM relies on mutual support at meetings, but unlike AA, the participants engage in cross talk, which is more like the exchanges that go on in professionally led therapy groups. Keith Humphreys, a leading researcher in the alcoholism field who is attuned to various kinds of alcohol problems, looked into whether the group was indeed attracting a segment of people who could moderate their drinking. He then reported on the characteristics of members.[30] Most all were white, employed, and college-educated.

A later study[31] looked at the computer-based MM format, comparing it with a version that was more highly structured. Both approaches turned out to be beneficial over time, even after a one-year follow up, with the structured version doing a bit better. This also reflects an emerging body of research on different ways that people can use computer programs to cut back on their drinking.

MM has achieved a reasonable measure of success, with meetings available in municipalities across the country. For example, as of this writing, there are three in New York, and one in Los Angeles. Interestingly though, MM posits that one has to start the program by abstaining from alcohol for thirty days. This latter point, ironically, may put off as many potential members as does AA's announced goal of abstinence; as for AA, one only needs "a desire to stop drinking." Many alcoholics have come to AA meetings while reluctant to stop drinking and have seated themselves at the back of the room, hoping to eventually get a handle on their problem. Whatever later ensues, their initial contacts can be helpful for them. Conversely, MM's website is informative to anyone wanting to limit their drinking.

NETWORK THERAPY

The approaches to alcoholism recovery we have discussed so far are based on people being helped without active input from their families or friends; yet if professional help is sought out, these sources of support can be brought in to play a valuable role. We have seen in AA how social support from people who were initially strangers can come to be helpful, so why not draw on people whom a person has known for many years? One might say that these people have previously been ignored, misled, or angrily put off, but there should be a way to make use of all those relationships and the concern inherent in them to help the afflicted person.

A variety of approaches that entail management by a therapist or a physician are now being used to treat alcoholics and drug addicts. There are also medications being used, with varying degrees of effectiveness, depending on the specific drug problem. Methadone and buprenorphine, for example, are maintenance drugs that are highly effective at blocking the effects of heroin and painkillers. What I would like to do here, however, is to illustrate how professionals use support from family and friends to help addicted people get better.

Many years ago, not long after I got out of psychiatric training, I got a federal grant to teach doctors about how to treat addiction. At that time, psychiatrists (including myself) had no systematic therapy to draw on for dealing with such patients. All we had available was to talk to them about their "underlying problems," or to tell them, "Go to AA, and come back when you've stopped drinking." I would like to explain why neither of these options seemed very effective.

I soon came to realize that once someone had become addicted to alcohol, the compulsion to drink was already long-established, and now operated independent of any previous conflict, insecurity, or anger that might have played a role in its origin. This was an important realization, because it became clear that addicted patients had to undergo some major transformation in their own outlooks and not just talk about their problem. Their problems were not like those of my depressed or anxious patients who could look back on how their troubles had started and, as it were, rewind that tape. On the other hand, AA did seem to have the ability to help some people experience the necessary transformation. But as for being told by the doctor to go AA, patients would often see this as a rejection, or an admission that the doctor had no solution for them anyway. They would usually go home and keep drinking.

But my grant designated me as a Career Teacher in Alcohol and Drug Abuse, and doctors around the medical school started referring their alcoholic patients to me. The patients were in enough denial that even the most willing of them could not convey the full nature of their drinking problem. In addition, they were unlike my other psychiatric patients who, when their symptoms got worse, would be all the more likely to come back to sessions hoping for relief. If the alcoholic patients slipped back into drinking, the denial of their illness would drive them to protect their drinking all the more, and they might stay home or even drop out of treatment.

Systemic family therapy was coming into acceptance at the time. It was an interesting approach, which I had learned about not long before as a resident in psychiatry. It was premised on the assumption that patients' problems were often embedded and fueled in the family's social system. The idea was to figure out how the drinking was expressing issues like anger between family members, or inability of the parents to properly manage their children. A therapist could then, with the right insight and talents, try to restructure relations among family members so that the symptom no longer had the pressure behind it, and it would abate. Sometimes the idea was simply to help people get along better together. This approach sometimes worked nicely. But it did not seem that one could restructure relations in a family to undo an addiction, given that the addiction had already established itself independent of family input. Instead, the role of the family or close, long-standing friends could be to support the patient's *own* ongoing initiative for recovery. Relationships among family members almost always improved when the patient stopped drinking, but not because the system was restructured. Rather, these patients were giving up a behavior that was like a cancer for all those around them.

Having family and close friends involved on an ongoing basis was also appealing because they could help to undermine the patient's denial. A wife would say, "But you have to tell the doctor about how you've gone to work late after you go out drinking." Family and friends can also support patients in staying sober, and leave them feeling that they have people behind them who care for them. The key point was that as a network—I called the approach Network Therapy[32]—they were much more effective than they could have been as individuals. The patient could not easily walk out on them all at once when they were supportive and not angry. The latter point, supportive but not angry, was all the more important if the patient had a slip and did drink. It was always important to maintain a caring tone. I would have to make this clear sometimes when it needed to be emphasized to an angry spouse or sibling.

As in AA and SMART Recovery, the objective here was abstinence, because Network Therapy was tailored for the truly addicted, when moderation was not something they could sustain. Network Therapy does borrow from AA the notion of being on the lookout for "people, places, and things" that can lead to drinking. Both patient and network would discuss where the vulnerabilities were and what was coming up, such as a party or a long weekend that represented the potential for a slip. The network members were sometimes more aware of these trigger situations than were the patients themselves.

One patient, John, illustrated this approach well. He decided to call me because, as he said, "I gotta get clean." He had been sniffing heroin on and off while in college, but for the last six months since graduating he found himself doing this twice a day. At a second session, he had his cousin join him at my request. Together, we assembled his uncle and two friends at an ensuing session for continuing support. John did not want to go to AA, but agreed to take naltrexone, a heroin-blocking agent, and to do so in front of one or another of his network members three times a week on a schedule we all set up.

He did well, with an understanding that he would also not drink for a year. (His brothers had terrible addiction problems, and his father was alcoholic.) As the year was coming to a close, John, the network, and I worked out a plan for him to see if he could drink in a controlled way, but no more than two beers a day, and he stuck with the plan. Ultimately, in sessions with me, he decided to cut out alcohol entirely, and he did so over the several years that I had contact with him.

John's network was invaluable to his treatment in a number of ways. It helped in monitoring the naltrexone (this was before one could get a monthly dose by injection). It supported his abstinence and he was appreciative of its help. His network worked out his trial of controlled drinking with him. He collaborated with his network to set up a mutual agreement that if the drinking got out of hand, he would go to AA.

In this way, we have looked at how the support of other people can help a person overcome an addiction problem. This is not to slight individual counseling, larger programs like the therapeutic communities, or medications that are being developed to curb addiction. Both patients and their caring family members can potentially make use of all these options. As with many other compromising diseases, the advice of a trusted doctor or clinic and thoughtful investigation on one's own are good starting points for seeking out the best help for a given person. The task of choosing the best approach is not easy, but it certainly merits careful consideration and acquiring knowledge of what options may be most suitable. One episode of treatment is often not enough for addiction. Sometimes many attempts are needed until remission is achieved.

CAN YOUR DOCTOR HELP YOU?

There are two ways your doctor can help. First, she can apply any of the approaches we have just described, but this entails being expert on how to work with addicted patients. The other is to send you to someone else who has experience in treating addiction. I would like to give you, the reader, a sense of the level of expertise needed among doctors to deal with such problems. The bad news is that very few are expert in this area. The good news, at least for the future, is that a growing number of physicians are now gaining this expertise.

Here is some background on this area of practice, relative to heroin, which in many respects is the most intractable of abused drugs. By the end of the 1960s, during the Nixon administration, street crime due to heroin addiction had become a major national issue. In order to address this, perhaps more as a law and order initiative than as one of medical concern, the federal government approved the establishment of tightly regulated clinics to dispense methadone as an effective replacement for heroin. Some thirty years later, in 2000, buprenorphine (Suboxone) was approved to be prescribed for addiction to heroin or painkillers, and this could be done by doctors in their office practice if they met certain training criteria. The advantage to this is that it could be done without the burden of a restrictive clinic structure.

Methadone and buprenorphine are medications that provide needed options for doctors in treating opioid dependence. They are drugs that many addicts are inclined to take and continue taking, because they are opioids, and thus addictive themselves. This means, if nothing else, that once someone starts taking these drugs, it is hard for them to get off them.

Who prescribes buprenorphine? About 3% of American doctors are certified to prescribe buprenorphine in their offices. For some it has become a significant part of their practices, as well as an important way to address the current epidemic of addiction to painkiller medications. Although these "maintenance" drugs can be effective in targeting opioid addiction, they have no utility for other drugs of abuse, including alcohol.

But then, who are the physicians who can address the other drugs, like alcohol? The level of expertise for this task is harder to come by. As of this writing, there are 5,700 medical addiction specialists who have been certified in the addiction subspecialty, about a half percent of all doctors. This cadre may be able to do some of the training needed for new physicians, but hardly enough to treat some 60 million American substance abusers. To this number of subspecialists one might add some portion of the 4% of doctors who are psychiatrists, but many, perhaps most, would not see themselves as having the same competency in treating addiction as they have for treating other mental health problems.

The good news relates to the growth of interest within the medical profession in addiction problems, and the educational resources now available to doctors. Membership in medical organizations dealing with addiction has consistently increased over the years, with some 4,000 now in the two leading societies. These societies also provide continuing education for the growing number of physicians at the conferences and trainings they run on this issue.

One's family doctor can draw on such colleagues as resources to help patients, and insurers are underwriting addiction treatment now, as federally mandated to be covered with parity to other medical illnesses. Independent outpatient programs are expanding as well. Insurers should be able to provide counseling resources, usually in the hands of psychologists, social workers, and counselors with expertise in substance use disorders, and this is generally coupled with referral to AA or NA when needed.

Various types of professional help are available for the substance abuser; some are alternatives to traditional Twelve Step involvement, others are complementary to it. Often, the principal barrier to getting help for these problems may be a lack of initiative on the part of the people who should be seeking it out, or their inability to sort out what would constitute appropriate help for them.

WHAT PHYSICIANS CAN PRESCRIBE

The use of medications for addicted people goes back in the late nineteenth century to the prescription of morphine to treat opium addicts, and in the early twentieth century to disulfirm (Antabuse) for alcoholics. (Disulfirm makes one feel sick if one takes it and then drinks.) The most widely used medications today, methadone and buprenorphine, are for opioid replacement, and these two agents have been valuable on a public health level in addressing heroin and painkiller addiction. They generally predominate over AA in prescribing for these addictions because the drug categories they address are so highly tenacious that Twelve Step programs and psychotherapeutic approaches, when applied alone, often result in relapse.

Other medications have been found to be helpful for other addiction syndromes. Most of these are directed at modifying the vulnerability to heavy drinking or relapse to alcoholism. Some examples of these are naltrexone (Revia), acamprosate (Campral), and gabapentin (Neurontin). Unlike AA, where evaluation research is hard to carry out, most of the validated experience with these medications involves their use in carefully structured, placebo-controlled studies. Results vary between studies, but by and large they yield some improvement in outcome. Like AA, they tend to work for some people, but not all.

Let's consider naltrexone, recommended as a daily medication. It was originally developed for blocking the effects of heroin, but based on consideration of its effect on neurotransmitters, it was tested for alcoholism treatment and approved for use for decreasing craving and relapse.[33] One way of measuring its effectiveness is what is called "the number needed to treat" (NNT), derived from a statistical analysis of data collected from well-controlled studies. This refers to how many patients one would need to prescribe the medication (vs. placebo) in order to get the effect desired for at least one of those patients. In order to get one person to avoid a return to drinking (compared with placebo), the NNT for naltrexone is twenty. This means that a doctor prescribing naltrexone rather than placebo would, statistically anyway, get 5% more of detoxified patients to stay sober than with a placebo.[34] This is not a very compelling recommendation for the medication's effectiveness.

Another problem with naltrexone, as with most other drugs used to treat addiction, is that people stop taking it after a while. This happens even in carefully monitored research projects. In one big federal study,[35] for example, a group of alcoholics were detoxified and started on either naltrexone or acamprosate, another anti-alcohol drug. Over half of them had stopped taking the medication before the end of the sixteen-week study period. We do not really know what the long-term benefit of this prescribing is in community-based practice.

Issues like this raise some interesting points about the disparity between the research community and the day-to-day experiences in doctors' offices, and they reveal the kind of obscure controversies one may encounter in the medical addiction field. One issue relates to researchers' complaints about why their findings are often ignored by treatment staff on the front lines. Many of the clinical scientists deride the doctors and clinics that do not prescribe naltrexone for their patients as being backward, and are frustrated that this medication is not more widely used.

But there are some other problems with their use. The studies conducted on them are carried out with counseling being provided along with the prescribing. Most all general physicians do not have a close tie to a counselor or a counseling program. This means that the NNT figures would only apply to a limited number of medical practices. This suggests the need for much better collaboration between the medical and counseling communities. In reality, this would be hard to achieve for most busy medical practices. We can only hope for a better way to address this in the future.

The problem of non-prescribing also relates to the structure of treatment programs, like public and privately run clinics. Frontline contacts with patients are almost always in the hands of non-physician therapists, such as counselors or social workers. Caseloads are large and coordination of counseling activities with part-time medical staff is hard to achieve, but without such cooperation, it is not feasible to implement a medication regimen. Additionally, counseling staff can devote only a limited amount of time to any specific aspect of their efforts with a given patient. Medications that have a clear and definitive clinical impact, like methadone or buprenorphine, are widely used, as in methadone clinics. Medications that may or may not have an impact on a given patient's addictive behavior will inevitably command less of the counselor's limited time.

Interestingly, there is another way of looking at the prescribing of such drugs for alcoholism. When one examines the studies on naltrexone, there is a sizable placebo effect.[36] That is to say, a doctor prescribing the drug will achieve a benefit that is not only due to the drug's physiologic effect, but also to its psychological impact on the patient. This enhances the clinical impact because patients respond to medication simply because a doctor wrote the prescription. This aspect of prescribing also can improve the impact of the doctor's advice for cutting back on alcohol. It also has a positive effect, however, on encouraging physicians to deal with their patients' drinking problems, as both doctors and their patients believe in pills. If physicians have a pill to prescribe, they will feel they have a role as a "real" physician. Fortunately, this psychology has led general physicians to view alcoholism more as a legitimate disease, and to pay more attention to their alcoholic patients' needs.

WHAT ABOUT TALK THERAPY?

The cognitive behavioral approach is the best researched among these therapies, and it is increasingly widely applied. It teaches the substance abusing person to recognize relapse triggers and to learn to surmount them. This approach is premised on experiences that all treating clinicians encounter with their addicted patients. One way to put it is that the vulnerability to relapse is associated with people, places, and things—to use AA terminology—that have previously coincided with their drinking. If they drank in a bar, the same sort of venue can be a trigger for drinking. Similarly, for the people they drank with, or for mood problems like sadness or loneliness. A disappointment can trigger drinking. The association may be obvious to patients, or they may have to learn about it through encounters with triggers they experience while in therapy.

One thing that is remarkable about this is that a long time can elapse from the time of exposure to a trigger to a later relapse, and the only part of the sequence that is apparent may be the relapse itself, with the intermediate steps remaining outside the patient's awareness. I learned about this in a vivid way early on while I was beginning to treat addicted people:

Evelyn was addicted to amphetamines. At times she would get these stimulants from her diet doctor, and at other times she would steal from the pharmacy her father owned. (Security over controlled substances was not as strict then as it is today.) I had been treating her for some months, and she was now drug-free. One day, she missed a session, and came in the next week shamefacedly telling me she had had a relapse. Here is a summary of how the episode played out, with the full course of the relapse process out of her awareness:

"Let's start by looking at where you took the pills."
"In my apartment."
"Had you been planning to take them?"
"No."
"Well, why did you take them, then?"
"My roommate left, and they were on my night table."
"Were you planning to take them then?"
"Not really. I just took them."
"Where did you get them?"
"I had gone to the diet doctor."
"Were you planning to get the pills from him so you could take them later?"
"Not really. I just thought it would be good to have them around if I ever needed them."
"But weren't you planning to take them?"
"Not really. I wasn't thinking about that."

We began to explore what might have brought on this sequence, which clearly reflected a process that was ongoing for some time *unbeknownst* to Evelyn. It emerged that she had had an argument with her boyfriend earlier that day, and she was quite upset about it. She had previously taken pills when she was upset, and the argument had triggered the whole entire sequence. Part of her therapy needed to be focused on how such distress was a trigger for her drug taking, and how she could recognize this vulnerability, and get clear in her mind what she had to do to actively avoid relapse in the future when something upset her.

EPILOGUE

The wording of AA's Steps is quite clear, but in practice people who encounter the fellowship can have very different experiences. In addition, research gives us average outcomes, but a given person is not an average. That is to say, there are many different ways the support of AA's members and its spirituality can play out for someone who first enters its meeting rooms, and it is hard to say how that will unfold. Given this, and given the "cunning" nature of addiction, it is not surprising that AA has come to be controversial.

Another issue contributes to controversies over AA nowadays. In its early years, the fellowship was all there was to help alcoholics survive their addiction, so that many of its early members came to view it as the definitive answer for all people with alcohol problems. This was the case because in those days many alcoholics, having nowhere to turn for help, would sink into a profoundly compromised state, hardly retrievable by means other than the fellowship. Today, however, we have approaches that can be applied to people with substance use disorders before they become severely compromised. For many such people, we intervene early in the course of the illness when it has not reached an unmanageable state. This makes many with addiction problems, particularly those attuned to medications or therapy, question why such an intensive approach is necessary. After all, addicted people are inclined to balk at what they see as a movement that entails considerable demands of time and commitment to become abstinent, particularly when they are ambivalent about stopping their drinking or drug use. Furthermore, AA and abstinence are not necessary for every person who drinks too much. Many people can modify their drinking habits and then limit their drinking, and do well. These are typically people without the most severe of alcohol problems.

These new circumstances can lead one to miss the point of AA's benefits. Most importantly, many people *are* profoundly addicted to alcohol or to the drugs for which we have no definitive treatments. Many would lose their families, jobs, even their lives, without a Twelve Step option available to them. There are also people for whom abstinence is the wisest option, even though they are not at a point at which they are in terrible shape, at least not yet; some involvement in AA can be invaluable in helping them get clarity on the merits of giving up alcohol and drugs entirely.

Professionals and treatment programs that maintain a Twelve Step orientation are increasingly finding that this approach is compatible with the variety of psychotherapeutic and pharmacologic approaches now available. What is now needed on the part of professionals and treatment programs and on the part of Twelve Step members themselves is a willingness to make use of this compatibility. This is an issue that I have worked to promote, and I will continue to do so.

So here is a word for those who want to help an addicted person, be they friends, relatives, or even doctors. The option of recommending a Twelve Step meeting raises issues that are often neglected. AA may seem to be a black box, with no consideration of how individualized any given person's experience can be. It may not be clear how AA can be relevant for a given person, and one can tell someone to "go to AA" with little understanding of how the fellowship can be combined with enlightened treatment, as it well can and should be. I certainly hope this book has shed some light on such opportunity for help.

And then, there are those who treat alcoholics. They can skirt questions that come up when a patient of theirs encounters AA, questions whose answers require experience and good judgment: Is a particular patient suitable for referral to AA or NA? How can one help a person see how their encounter with the fellowship can be relevant and useful to them? Should they be pressed to get a sponsor? There are certainly no textbook-based answers to these questions.

One remarkable aspect of the Twelve Step experience that we have discussed in this book bears mention in closing. It illustrates how an intensely felt experience in the setting of AA membership can be transformative in a way that is quite different from what one may derive from psychotherapy or medications. Many long-established AA members who have achieved respite in the fellowship have undergone personal a transformation in a way that is different from the usual ways people arrive at rationally grounded changes. What can happen to them is what AA calls a spiritual awakening. This intense experience of belief and emotional change can leave a person quite different and rejuvenated in the many ways that we have discussed. Most notably, many of these people who were victims of craving for alcohol or drugs report that they are plagued by this no more; they can go on with their daily lives at peace without that compulsion. The profound effect of mutual support combined with a spiritual message can change people in ways that we cannot yet fully understand or predict.

NOTES

INTRODUCTION
1. Kaskutas et al. 2008.
2. M. Galanter and L. A. Kaskutas 2008.
3. *The Player*, 1992.
4. Alcoholics Anonymous. Tradition 12.
5. Alcoholics Anonymous. http://www.aa.org/.

CHAPTER 1
1. Alcoholics Anonymous 1957.
2. W. White 2014.
3. Alcoholics Anonymous World Services 2013.
4. M. D. Peterson and R. C. Vaughn (Eds.) 1988.
5. W. James 1929.
6. Alcoholics Anonymous World Services 2001, p. 567.
7. Alcoholics Anonymous World Services 2013, p. 9.
8. M. Weber 1947.
9. N. Robertson 2000.
10. A. Orange 2014.
11. Jonas et al. 2014.

CHAPTER 2
Questions About God and a Higher Power
1. W. White 2014.
2. Alcoholics Anonymous 2001, p. 63.
3. Alcoholics Anonymous 2001, p. 55.

So, Controversy Persists
1. Alcoholics Anonymous, 2001 p. 58.
2. M. Kolb and M. S. Propper 1976.
3. M. Ferri and M. Davoli 2006.
4. Project MATCH Research Group 1998.
5. D. Donovan and A. S. Floyd 2008.
6. R. H. Moos and B. S. Moos 2006.
7. L. Dodes and Z. Dodes 2013.
8. D. McIntire 2000.
9. R. H. Moos and B. S. Moos 2006.

10. K. Humphreys and R. H. Moos 2007.
11. R. Stinchfield and P. Owen 1998.
12. C. P. O'Brien 2015.
13. D. E. Jonas et al. 2014.
14. B. A. Johnson 2010.

Perceptions of Addiction
1. Alcoholics Anonymous 2001, p. 30.
2. American Psychiatric Association 1968.
3. A. T. McLellan et al. 2000.
4. H. Smith 1984.
5. M. L. Schrad 2011.
6. D. Zaridze et al. 2009.
7. S. Fedun 2014.
8. I. Ladegaard 2012.
9. Alcoholics Anonymous World Services 1965, p. 5.
10. A. Wikler 1971.
11. Alcoholics Anonymous 2001.
12. M. Galanter 1983 (b).
13. L. Wurmser 1978.
14. L. Dodes 2013.
15. American Psychiatric Association 1968.
16. American Psychiatric Association 1980.
17. American Psychiatric Association 1994.
18. American Psychiatric Association 2013.
19. M. Fox 2011.
20. E. E. Bouchery et al. 2011.
21. R. Saitz 2010.
22. G. Vaillant 1983.
23. A. Freud 1964.
24. M. J. Farah 2014.
25. F. A. Kozel 2005.
26. K. S. LaBar and R. Cabeza 2006.
27. B. A. Kuhl et al. 2007.
28. W. Jiang et al. 2013.

CHAPTER 3
1. M. Galanter et al. 2012.
2. M. Galanter et al. 2013 (c).
3. M. Galanter et al. 2013 (a).
4. M. Galanter et al. 2013 (b).
5. M. Galanter et al. 2014.
6. L. M. Najavits et al. 2013.
7. R. H. Moos and B. S. Moos et al. 2006.
8. A. Comte et al. 2009.
9. J. Bruner 1990.

CHAPTER 4
1. M. Galanter 1978.
2. M. Galanter and P. Buckley 1978.

3. M. Galanter et al. 1979.
4. M. Galanter 1983 (a).
5. M. Galanter 1997.
6. W. James 1929, p. 14.
7. H. H. Kelley 1967.
8. M. Fisher 2007.

CHAPTER 5

1. Alcoholics Anonymous 1965, p. 35.
2. Alcoholics Anonymous 2001, p. 63.
3. W. Miller and J. Baca 2001.
4. Alcoholics Anonymous World Services 1965, p. 21.
5. Alcoholics Anonymous World Services 1965, p. 25.
6. R. Lifton 1961.
7. L. Rambo and S. Bauman 2012.
8. W. White 2014, p. 176.
9. St. Augustine 1838.
10. M. Horowitz 1956.
11. S. Hymer 1995.
12. E. Todd 1985.
13. C. Kratz 1991.
14. K. Pype 2011.
15. C. Kratz 1991.
16. K. Pype 2011.
17. J. Silk 1998.
18. M. Bosworth 2002.
19. C. Pansera and J. La Guardia 2012.
20. Alcoholics Anonymous 2001, p. 63.
21. Alcoholics Anonymous World Services 2001, p. 76.
22. E. Sifton 2003.
23. Alcoholics Anonymous World Services 1965, p. 96.
24. W. James 1929, p. 454.
25. W. James 1929, p. 371.
26. S. Post 2014.
27. J. Adler et al. 2005.
28. R. J. Foster 1992.
29. B. Spilka et al. 1985.
30. M. Galanter et al. 1991.
31. R. Coles 1990.
32. T. M. Luhrman 2012.
33. T. M. Luhrman 2012, p. 133.
34. Alcoholics Anonymous 2001, p. 94.
35. D. P. Rice 1995.
36. R. B. Huebner and L. W. Kantor 2011.
37. Center on Addiction and Substance Abuse, Columbia University 1994.
38. M. Weber 1947.
39. K. Makela et al. 1996.
40. Alcoholics Anonymous World Services 1965.
41. Alcoholics Anonymous World Services 2013.
42. Alcoholics Anonymous World Services 2013.

43. International Doctors in Alcoholics Anonymous 2011.
44. M. Galanter et al. 1990.

CHAPTER 6

1. P. J. P. Whelan et al. 2009.
2. F. Riessman 1965.
3. O. H. Mowrer 1964.
4. B. T. King and I. L. Janis 1956.
5. Alcoholics Anonymous 2001, p. 94.
6. M. E. Pagano et al. 2004.
7. B. L Crape et al. 2002.
8. J. J. Viola et al. 2009.
9. S. L. Brown et al. 2003.
10. M. E. Kahn and C. Fua 1992.
11. K. Vick 2005.
12. R. C. Kessler et al. 2001.
13. R. Kohn et al. 2004.
14. J. L. Goldstein and M. M. L. Godemont 2003.
15. J. Gray et al. 2001.
16. A. Stimpson et al. 2013.
17. S. Shinde et al. 2013.
18. E. G. Poser 1966.
19. H. H. Strupp and S. W. Hadley 1979.
20. J. S. Tonigan and S. L. Rice 2010.
21. J. D. Frank and J. B. Frank 1961.

CHAPTER 7

1. Alcoholics Anonymous 1957.
2. L. A. Kaskutas et al. 2005.
3. M. Galanter et al. 2013(c).
4. M. Galanter et al. 2012
5. M. Galanter et al. 2013(a).
6. L. A. Festinger 1957.

CHAPTER 8

1. R. Putnam 2001.
2. M. Galanter 1999.
3. Garcia et al. 2015.

CHAPTER 9

1. M. Ferri and M. Davoli 2006.
2. S. Magura 2013.
3. M. S. Subbaraman and L. A. Kaskutas 2012.
4. N. Robertson 2000.
5. P. Ryberg 2001.
6. M. Galanter et al. 1990.
7. D. McDowell et al. 1996.
8. L. Goldfarb et al. 1996.
9. A. Van Zee 2009.
10. R. D. Weiss et al. 2011.

11. G. E. Woody et al. 2008.
12. Narcotics Anonymous World Services 2007.

CHAPTER 10
1. W. White 2014.
2. M. Weber 1947.
3. R. Stinchfield and P. Owen 1998.
4. L. Keso and M. Salaspuro 1990.
5. P. Haldeman 2013.
6. U. S. News 2014.
7. C. Silberstein et al. 1996.
8. S. M. Taylor et al. 1997.

CHAPTER 11
1. T. S. Kuhn 1962.
2. E. O. Wilson 1975.
3. R. Descartes 1641.
4. I. Fried et al. 1997.
5. C. Darwin 1871/2004.
6. C. Darwin 1871/2004. p. 325.
7. K. Lorenz 1974.
8. M. Galanter 1978
9. W. D. Hamilton 1975.
10. R. L. Trivers 1971.
11. A. Jolly 1972
12. S. J. Suomi et al. 1976.
13. B. G. Campbell 1974.
14. D. Pilbeam 1972.
15. R. I. M. Dunbar 1998.
16. H. Damasio et al. 1994.
17. E. Herrmann et al. 2007.
18. M. Galanter 2014.
19. N. D. Volkow et al. 2007.
20. J. T. Cacioppo and G. G. Bernston 2004.
21. G. Rizzolatti and M. Fabbri-Destro 2010.
22. A. Bateman and P. Fonagy 2006.
23. M. V. Lombardo et al. 2010.
24. G. Hein et al. 2010.
25. R. Descartes 1641.
26. V. E. Stone and P. Gerrans 2006.
27. J. Zaki and K. N. Ochsner 2006.
28. R. N. Spreng and R. A. Mar 2012.
29. C. Pennartz 2011.
30. K. Foerde and D. Shohamy 2011.
31. R. J. Lifton 1961.
32. J. Piaget and P. Kegan 1929.
33. I. Fried et al. 1997.
34. S. H. Wang et al. 2012.
35. M. Koenigs et al. 2007.
36. A. Javanbakht 2011.

37. H. Kober et al. 2010.
38. H. Markus et al. 1982.
39. H. Markus et al. 1982.
40. M. G. Swora 2002.
41. D. I. Tamir and J. P. Mitchell 2012.
42. C. E. Forbes and J. Grafman 2010.
43. L. Festinger 1957.
44. J. Kerns et al. 2004.
45. V. Van Veen et al. 2009.
46. H. D. Critchley 2005.
47. M. Galanter and S. G. Post 2014.
48. T. S. Kuhn 1962.
49. G. Hein et al. 2010.
50. Alcoholics Anonymous 2001, p. 63.
51. M. Galanter et al., in press.
52. J. A. McGeoch 1933.
53. M. E. Bouton 2004.

CHAPTER 12

1. G. Glaser 2015.
2. L. Dodes and Z. Dodes 2013.
3. C. P. O'Brien 2015.
4. B. A. Johnson 2014.
5. J. Nowinski et al. 1992.
6. Project MATCH Research Group 1998.
7. R. Longabaugh et al. 1998.
8. J. F. Kelly & C. Greene 2014.
9. J. F. Kelly et al. 2006.
10. M. Galanter et al. 2008.
11. L. A. Kaskutas 2009.
12. J. S. Mausner and S. Kramer 1985.
13. R. H. Moos and B. S. Moos 2006.
14. R. H. Moos and B. S. Moos 2006.
15. G. J. Connors et al. 2001.
16. K. Humphreys et al. 2014.
17. C. D. Emrick et al. 1993.
18. G. E. Vaillant 1995.
19. A. R. Krentzman et al. 2012.
20. K. Humphreys et al. 1999.
21. J. S. Tonigan et al. 2001.
22. C. Timko et al. 2000.
23. R. Fiorentine et al. 2000.
24. J. McKellar et al. 2003.
25. W. C. Moyer 2007.
26. S. M. Gilman et al. 2001.
27. L. M. Glickman et al. 2005.
28. The Betty Ford Institute Consensus Panel 2007.
29. L. A. Kaskutas and L. A. Ritter 2015.

CHAPTER 13

1. Narcotics Anonymous World Services, www.na.org.
2. M. Galanter et al. 2013 (b).
3. Narcotics Anonymous World Services 1998.
4. W. L. White 2014.
5. W. L. White 2014.
6. Narcotics Anonymous World Services 2008.
7. M. Galanter et al. 2013 (a).
8. M. Galanter et al. 2014.
9. L. M. Najavits and D. Hien 2013.
10. D. A. Dawson et al. 2006.
11. AA Agnostica, aaagnostica.org.
12. Alcoholics Anonymous 1957.
13. E. Kurtz 1979.
14. R. C. 2014.
15. E. Kurtz 1979.
16. R. C. 2012.
17. Alcoholics Anonymous World Services 2014, p. 7.
18. L. S. 2006.
19. T. Jacobs-Stewart 2010.
20. D. Rode 2012.
21. D. Rode, http://12steppathtoenlightenment.com/dorena.htm.
22. A. Ellis 2004.
23. A. Beck 2008.
24. J. Trimpey 1995.
25. SMART Recovery 2014.
26. A. Kishline and S. Maloy 2007.
27. National Institute on Alcohol Abuse and Alcoholism
28. National Institute on Alcohol Abuse and Alcoholism 2015.
29. M. Solomon 2005.
30. K. Humphreys and E. Klaw 2001.
31. R. Hester et al. 2011.
32. M. Galanter 1993.
33. J. R. Volpicelli et al. 1992.
34. D. E. Jonas et al. 2014.
35. R. L. Stout et al. 2014.
36. J. Chick et al. 2000.

REFERENCES

Adler, J., Underwood, A., Whitford, B., Chung, J., Juarez, V., Bervett, D., Lorraine, A. In search of the spiritual. Newsweek 146:46–64, 2005.

Alcoholics Anonymous [Website]. http://www.aa.org/

AA Agnostica: A Space for AA agnostics, atheists, and freethinkers worldwide [Website]. http://aaagnostica.org/

Alcoholics Anonymous. The Big Book. 4th ed. New York, NY: AA World Services, 2001.

Alcoholics Anonymous. Alcoholics Anonymous Comes of Age. New York, NY: Alcoholics Anonymous Publishing, 1957.

Alcoholics Anonymous World Services. Alcoholics Anonymous: The Story of How Many Thousands of Men and Women Have Recovered from Alcoholism. 4th ed. New York, NY: Alcoholics Anonymous Publishing, 2001.

Alcoholics Anonymous World Services. Many Paths to Spirituality [Pamphlet]. New York, NY: Alcoholics Anonymous Publishing, 2014.

Alcoholics Anonymous World Services. The AA Service Manual Combined with Twelve Concepts for World Service. New York, NY: Alcoholics Anonymous Publishing, 2013.

Alcoholics Anonymous World Services. The AA Member-Medications and Other Drugs [Pamphlet]. New York, NY: Alcoholics Anonymous Publishing, 2011 (Originally published 1984).

Alcoholics Anonymous World Services. Twelve Steps and Twelve Traditions. New York, NY: Alcoholics Anonymous Publishing, 1965.

American Psychiatric Association. Desk Reference to the Diagnostic and Statistical Manual of Mental Disorders, 5th. Edition. Washington, DC: American Psychiatric Association, 2013.

American Psychiatric Association. Diagnostic and Statistical Manual of Mental Disorders, 2nd. Edition. Arlington, VA: American Psychiatric Publishing, 1968.

American Psychiatric Association. Diagnostic and Statistical Manual of Mental Disorders, 3rd. Edition. Arlington, VA: American Psychiatric Publishing, 1980.

American Psychiatric Association. Diagnostic and Statistical Manual of Mental Disorders, 4th. Edition. Washington, DC: American Psychiatric Association, 1994.

American Psychiatric Association. Diagnostic and Statistical Manual of Mental Disorders, 5th. Edition. Arlington, VA: American Psychiatric Publishing, 2013.

Augustine, St. The Confessions of St. Augustine (E. B. Pusey, Trans.). Oxford, England: J. H. Parker, 1838.

Bateman, A., Fonagy, P. Mentalization. New York, NY: Oxford University Press, 2006.

Beck, A. T. The evolution of the cognitive model of depression and its neurobiological correlates. American Journal of Psychiatry 165(8):969–977, 2008.

Bouchery, E. E., Harwood, H. J., Sacks, J. J., Simon, C. J., Brewer, R. D. Economic costs of excessive alcohol consumption in the U.S., 2006. American Journal of Prevention Medicine 41:516–524, 2011.

Bouton, M. E. Context and behavioural processes in extinction. Learning and Memory 11(5):485–494.

Bosworth, M. The U. S. Federal Prison System. California, London, New Delhi: Sage Publications, 2002.

Brown, S. L., Nesse, R. M., Vinokur, A. D., Smith, D. Providing social support may be more beneficial than receiving it: Results from a prospective study of mortality. Psychological Science 14(4):320–327, 2003.

Bruner, J. Acts of Meaning. Cambridge: Harvard University Press, 1990.

C., R. A History of Agnostic Groups in AA. Canada: AA Agnostica, 2012.

C., R. Don't Tell: Stories and Essays by Agnostics and Atheists in AA. Canada: AA Agnostica, 2014.

Cacioppo, J. T., Berntson, G. G. Essays in Social Neuroscience. Cambridge, MA: MIT Press, 2004.

Campbell, B. G. Human Evolution: Introduction to Man's Adaptations. Chicago: Aldine, 1974.

Canagasaby, A., Vinson, D. C. Screening for hazardous or harmful drinking using one or two quantity–frequency questions. Alcohol and Alcoholism 40:208–213, 2005.

Chick, J., Anton, R., Checinski, K., Croop, R., Drummond, D. C., Farmer, R., Labriola, D., Marshall, J., Moncrieff, J., Morgan, M. Y. A multicentre, randomized, double-blind, placebo-controlled trial of naltrexone in the treatment of alcohol dependence or abuse. Alcohol and Alcoholism 35(6):587–593, 2000.

Center on Addiction and Substance Abuse. The cost of substance abuse to America's health care system; Report 2: Medicare hospital costs, 1994. Retrieved from http://www.casacolumbia.org/addiction-research/reports/cost-substance-abuse-america's-health-care-system-report-2-medicare

Coles, R. The Spiritual Life of Children. Boston: Houghton Mifflin, 1990.

Comte, A., Bridges, J. A General View of Positivism. Cambridge, England: Cambridge University Press, 2009.

Connors, G. J., Tonigan, J. S., Miller, W. R. A longitudinal model of intake symptomatology, AA participation and outcome: retrospective study of the project MATCH outpatient and aftercare samples. Journal of Studies on Alcohol and Drugs 62(6):817–825, 2001.

Crape, B. L., Latkin, C. A., Laris, A. S., Knowlton, A. R. The effects of sponsorship in 12-step treatment of injection drug users. Drug and Alcohol Dependence 65(3):291–301, 2002.

Critchley, H. D. Neural mechanisms of autonomic, affective, and cognitive integration. Journal of Comparative Neurology 493(1):154–166, 2005.

Damasio, H., Grabowski, T., Frank, R., Galaburda, A. M., Damasio, A. R. The return of Phineas Gage: Clues about the brain from the skull of a famous patient. Science 264(5162):1102–1105, 1994.

Darwin, C. The Descent of Man. Digireads.com Publishing, 2004. (Originally published in 1871).

Dawson, D. A., Grant, B. F., Stinson, F. S., Chou, P. S. Maturing out of alcohol dependence: The impact of transitional life events. Journal of Studies on Alcohol 67(2):195–203, 2006.

Descartes, R. Meditations on First Philosophy. (A. Bailey, Ed.) (I. Johnson, Trans.). Peterborough, Ontario, Canada: Broadview Press, 2013 (Originally published in 1641).

Dodes, L., Dodes, Z. The Sober Truth. Boston, MA: Beacon Press, 2013.

Donovan, D., Floyd, A. S. Facilitating involvement in Twelve-Step programs. In Galanter, M. and Kaskutas, L. A. (Eds.) Recent Developments in Alcoholism. New York, NY: Springer, 2008, pp. 309–311.

Dunbar, R. I. M. The social brain hypothesis. Evolutionary Anthropology: Issues, News, and Reviews 6(5):178–190, 1998.

Ellis, A. Rational Emotive Behavioral Therapy: It Works for Me—It Can Work for You. Amherst, NY: Prometheus Books, 2004.

Emrick C. D., Tonigan, J. S., Montgomery, H., et al. Alcoholics Anonymous: What is currently known? In Research on Alcoholics Anonymous: Opportunities and Alternatives, Edited by McCrady, B. S., Miller, W. R. New Brunswick, NJ, Rutgers Center of Alcohol Studies, 1993, pp. 41–76.

Ewing, J. A. Detecting alcoholism, the CAGE questionnaire. Journal of the American Medical Association 252:1905–1907, 1984.

Farah, M. J., Hutchinson, J. B., Phelps, E. A., Wagner, A. D. Functional MRI-based lie detection: scientific and societal challenges. Nature Reviews Neuroscience 15:123–131, 2014.

Fedun, S. How alcohol conquered Russia. The Atlantic. September 25, 2013.

Ferri, M., Davoli, M. Alcoholics Anonymous and other 12-step programmes for alcohol dependence (review). Cochrane Database of Systematic Reviews 3:1–25, 2006.

Festinger, L. A. A Theory of Cognitive Dissonance. Stanford, CA: Stanford University Press, 1957.

Fiorentine, R., Hillhouse, M. P. Drug treatment and 12-step program participation: The additive effects of integrated recovery activities. Journal of Substance Abuse Treatment 18, 65–74, 2000.

Fisher, M. Seeking recovery, finding confusion. The Washington Post, July 22, 2007.

Foerde, K., Shohamy, D. The role of the basal ganglia in learning and memory: Insight from Parkinson's disease. Neurobiology of Learning and Memory 96(4):624–636, 2011.

Forbes, C. E., Grafman, J. The role of the human prefrontal cortex in social cognition and moral judgment. Annual Review of Neuroscience 33:299–324, 2010.

Foster, R. J. Prayer: Finding the Heart's True Home. San Francisco, CA: Harper, 1992.

Fox, M. CDC: Alcohol abuse costs U.S. $224 billion a year. National Journal, October 17, 2011. Retrieved from http://www.nationaljournal.com/healthcare/cdc-alcohol-abuse-costs-u-s-224-billion-a-year-20111017.

Frank, J. D., Frank, J. B. Persuasion and Healing: A Comparative Study of Psychotherapy. Baltimore, MD: Johns Hopkins University Press, 1961.

Freud, A. The ego and mechanisms of defense. New York, NY: International University Press, 1964.

Fried, I., MacDonald, K. A., Wilson, C. A. Single neuron activity in human hippocampus and amygdala during recognition of faces and objects. Neuron 18:753–765, 1997.

Galanter, M. The "relief effect": A sociobiologic model for neurotic distress and large group therapy. American Journal of Psychiatry 135:588–591, 1978.

Galanter, M. Engaged "Moonies": The impact of a charismatic group on adaptation and behavior. Archives of General Psychiatry 40:1197–1202, 1983. (a)

Galanter, M. Psychotherapy for alcohol and drug abuse: An approach based on learning theory. Journal of Psychiatric Treatment and Evaluation 5:551–556, 1983. (b)

Galanter, M. Network Therapy for Alcohol and Drug Abuse: A New Approach in Practice. New York, NY: Basic Books (HarperCollins), 1993.

Galanter, M. Spiritual recovery movements and contemporary medical care. Psychiatry: Interpersonal and Biological Processes 60:236–248, 1997.

Galanter, M. Cults: Faith, Healing, and Coercion. 2nd ed. Oxford and New York: Oxford University Press, 1999.

Galanter, M. Alcoholics Anonymous and twelve-step recovery: A model based on social and cognitive neuroscience. The American Journal on Addictions 23: 300–307, 2014.

Galanter, M., Buckley P. Evangelical religion and meditation: psychotherapeutic effects. Journal of Nervous and Mental Disease 166:685–691, 1978.

Galanter, M., Dermatis, H., Post, S., Sampson, C. Spirituality-based recovery from drug addiction in the twelve-step fellowship of Narcotics Anonymous. Journal of Addiction Medicine 7:189–195, 2013.

Galanter, M., Dermatis, H., Post, S., Santucci, C. Abstinence from drugs of abuse in community-based members of Narcotics Anonymous. Journal of Studies on Alcohol and Drugs 74:349–352, 2013. (a)

Galanter, M., Dermatis, H., Sampson, C. Narcotics Anonymous: A comparison of military veterans and non-veterans 33:1–9, 2014. (b)

Galanter, M., Dermatis, H., Santucci, C. Young people in Alcoholics Anonymous: The role of spiritual orientation and AA member affiliation. Journal of Addictive Diseases 31:173–182, 2012.

Galanter, M., Dermatis, H., Stanievich, J., Santucci, C. Physicians in long-term recovery who are members of Alcoholics Anonymous. The American Journal on Addictions 22:323–328, 2013. (c)

Galanter, M., Josipovic, Z., Dermatis, H., Weber, J., Millard, M. A. Neural correlates of prayer in members of Alcoholics Anonymous: An fMRI study [In Press].

Galanter M., Kaskutas, L. A. Recent Developments in Alcoholism, Vol. XVIII. Research on Alcoholics Anonymous and Spirituality in Addiction Recovery. New York, NY: Kluwer/Plenum Press, 2008.

Galanter, M., Larson, D., Rubenstone, E. Christian psychiatry: The impact of evangelical belief on clinical practice. The American Journal of Psychiatry 148:90–95, 1991.

Galanter, M., Post, S. G., Eds. Special Issue: Alcoholics Anonymous: New directions in research on spirituality and recovery. Alcoholism Treatment Quarterly 32(2–3), 2014.

Galanter, M., Rabkin R., Rabkin J., Deutsch A. The "Moonies": A psychological study. American Journal of Psychiatry 136:165–170, 1979.

Galanter, M., Talbott, D., Gallegos, K., Rubenstone, E. Combined Alcoholics Anonymous and professional care for addicted physicians. American Journal of Psychiatry 147:64–68, 1990.

Garcia, A., Anderson, B., Humphreys, K. Fourth and fifth step groups: A new and growing self-help organization for underserved Latinos with substance use disorders. Alcoholism Treatment Quarterly 33(2):1–9, 2015.

Gilman, S. M., Galanter, M., Dermatis, H. Methadone anonymous: A 12-step program for methadone maintained heroin addicts. Substance Abuse 22: 247–256, 2001.

Glaser, G. The false gospel of Alcoholics Anonymous. The Atlantic, April 2015.

Glickman, L., Galanter, M., Dermatis, H., Dingle, S., Hall, L. Pathways to Recovery. Journal of Maintenance in the Addictions 2:77–90, 2005.

Goldfarb, L., Galanter, M., McDowell, D., Lifshutz, H., Dermatis, H. Medical student and patient attitudes toward religion and spirituality in the recovery process. The American Journal of Drug and Alcohol Abuse 22:549–561, 1996.

Goldstein, J., Godemont, M. L. The legend and lessons of Geel, Belgium: A 1500-year-old legend, a 21st-century model. Community Mental Health Journal 39(5):441–458, 2003.

Gray, J., Spurway, P., McClatchey, M. Lay therapy intervention with families at risk for parenting difficulties: The Kempe Community Caring Program. Child Abuse & Neglect 25(5):641–655, 2001.

Haldeman, P. An intervention for Malibu. The New York Times: ST1, September 3, 2013.

Hamilton, W. D. Innate social aptitudes of man: An approach from evolutionary genetics. In R. Fox (Ed.) Biosocial Anthropology. New York, NY: John Wiley & Sons, 1975, pp. 133–155.

Hein, G., Silani, G., Preuschoff, K., Batson, C. D., Singer, T. Neural responses to ingroup and outgroup members' suffering predict individual differences in costly helping. Neuron 68:149–160, 2010.

Herrmann, E., Call, J., Hernàndez-Lloreda, M. V., Hare, B., Tomasello, M. Humans have evolved specialized skills of social cognition: The cultural intelligence hypothesis. Science 317(5843):1360–1366, 2007.

Hester, R. K., Delaney, H. D., Campbell, W. ModerateDrinking.Com and moderation management: Outcomes of a randomized clinical trial with non-dependent problem drinkers. Journal of Consulting and Clinical Psychology 79(2):215–224, 2011.

Horowitz, M. W. The psychology of confession. The Journal of Criminal Law, Criminology, and Police Science 47:197–204, 1956.

Huebner, R. B., Kantor, L. W. Advances in alcoholism treatment. Alcohol Research & Health: the Journal of the National Institute on Alcohol Abuse and Alcoholism 33:295–299, 2011.

Humphreys, K., Huebsch, P. D., Finney, J. W., Moos, R. H. A Comparative evaluation of substance abuse treatment: V. substance abuse treatment can enhance the effectiveness of self-help groups. Alcoholism: Clinical and Experimental Research 23: 558–563, 1999.

Humphreys, K., Klaw, E. Can targeting nondependent problem drinkers and providing Internet-based services expand access to assistance for alcohol problems? A study of the Moderation Management self-help/mutual aid organization. Journal of Studies on Alcohol and Drugs 62(4):528, 2001.

Humphreys, K., Moos, R. H. Encouraging posttreatment self-help group involvement to reduce demand for continuing care services: Two-year clinical and utilization outcomes. Alcoholism: Clinical & Experimental Research 26:151–158, 2007.

Hymer, S. Therapeutic and redemptive aspects of religious confession. Journal of Religion and Health 34:41–54, 1995.

IMS: SDI's Total Patient Tracker (TPT), Projected Patient Count, Moving Annual Total 2003–2013.

International Doctors in Alcoholics Anonymous. (2011). www.idaa.org

Jacobs-Stewart, T. Mindfulness and the 12 Steps. Center City, MN: Hazelden Publishing, 2010.

Javanbakht, A. A neural network model for schemas based on pattern completion. Journal of the American Academy of Psychoanalysis and Dynamic Psychiatry 39(2):243–261, 2011.

James, W. The Varieties of Religious Experience. New York, NY: Modern Library, 1929.

Jiang, W., Liu, H., Liao, J., Ma, X., Rong, P., Tang, Y., Wang, W. A functional MRI study of deception among offenders with antisocial personality disorders. Neuroscience 244:90–98, 2013.

Johnson, B. A. Why rehab doesn't work. Dallas News. November 26, 2010.

Jolly, A. The Evolution of Primate Behavior. New York, NY: Macmillan, 1972.

Jonas, D. E., Amick, H. R., Feltner, C. Bobashev, G., Thomas, K., Wines, R., Kim, M. M., Shanahan, E., Gass, E., Rowe, C. J., Garbutt, J. C. Pharmacotherapy for adults with alcohol use disorders in outpatient settings: A systematic review and meta-analysis. Journal of the American Medical Association 311:1889–1900, 2014.

Kahn, M. W., Fua, C. Counselor training as a treatment for alcoholism: The helper therapy principle in action. International Journal of Social Psychiatry 38(3): 208–214, 1992.

Kaskutas, L. A. Alcoholics Anonymous effectiveness: Faith meets science. Journal of Addictive Diseases 28(2):145–57, 2009.

Kaskutas, L. A., Ritter, L. A. Consistency between beliefs and behavior regarding use of substances in recovery. Sage Open 5(1), 2015.

Kelley, H. H. Attribution theory in social psychology. In D. Levine (Ed.) Nebraska Symposium on Motivation, Vol XV. Lincoln, NE: University of Nebraska Press, 1967, pp. 192–238.

Kelly, J. F., Greene, M. C. Toward an enhanced understanding of the psychological mechanisms by which spirituality aids recovery in Alcoholics Anonymous. Alcoholism Treatment Quarterly 32(2–3):299–318, 2014.

Kelly, J. F., Stout, R., Zywiak, W., Schneider, R. A 3-year study of addiction mutual-help group participation following intensive outpatient treatment. Alcoholism: Clinical and Experimental Research 30(8):1381–1392, 2006.

Kerns, J. G., Cohen, J. D., MacDonald, A. W., Cho, R. Y., Stenger, V. A., Carter, C. S. Anterior cingulate conflict monitoring and adjustments in control. Science 303(5660):1023–1026, 2004.

Keso, L., Salaspuro, M. Inpatient treatment of employed alcoholics: A randomized clinical trial on Hazelden-type and traditional treatment. Alcoholism: Clinical and Experimental Research 14:584–589, 1990.

Kessler, R. C., Berglund, P. A., Bruce, M. L., Koch, J. R., Laska, E. M., Leaf, P. J., Manderscheid, R. W., ... Wang, P. S. The prevalence and correlates of untreated serious mental illness. Health Services Research 36(6 Pt 1):987–1007, 2001.

King, B. T., Janis, I. L. Comparison of the effectiveness of improvised versus non-improvised role-playing in producing opinion changes. Human Relations 9: 177–186, 1956.

Kishline, A., Maloy, S. Face to Face: A Deadly Drunk Driver, a Grieving Young Mother, and Their Astonishing True Story of Tragedy and Forgiveness. New York, NY: Meredith Books, 2007.

Kober, H., Mende-Siedlecki, P., Kross, E. F., Weber, J., Mischel, W., Hart, C. L., Ochsner, K. N. Prefrontal–striatal pathway underlies cognitive regulation of craving. Proceedings of the National Academy of Sciences 107(33):14811–14816, 2010.

Koenigs, M., Young, L., Adolphs, R., Tranel, D., Cushman, F., Hauser, M., Damasio, A. Damage to the prefrontal cortex increases utilitarian moral judgments. Nature 446(7138):908–911, 2007.

Kohn, R., Saxena, S., Levav, I., Saraceno, B. The treatment gap in mental health care. Bulletin of the World Health Organization 82:858–866, 2004.

Kozel, F. A., Johnson, K. A., Mu, Q., Grenesko, E. L., Laken, S. J., George, M. S. Detecting deception using functional magnetic resonance imaging. Biological Psychiatry 58:605–613, 2005.

Kratz, C. Amusement and absolution: Transforming narratives during confession of social debts. American Anthropologist 93:826–851, 1991.

Krentzman, A. R., Brower, K. J., Cranford, J. A., Bradley, J. C., Robinson, E. A. Gender and extroversion as moderators of the association between Alcoholics Anonymous and sobriety. Journal of Studies on Alcohol and Drugs 73(1):44–52, 2012.

Kuhl, B. A., Dudukovic, N. M., Kahn, I., Wagner, A. D. Decreased demands on cognitive control reveal the neural processing benefits of forgetting. Nature Neuroscience 10:908–914, 2007.

Kuhn, T. S. The Structure of Scientific Revolutions. Chicago, IL: University of Chicago Press, 1962.

Kurtz, E. Not-God: A History of Alcoholics Anonymous. Center City, MN: Hazelden Publishing, 1979.

LaBar, K. S., Cabeza, R. (2006). Cognitive neuroscience of emotional memory. Nature Reviews Neuroscience 7:54–64, 2006.

Ladegaard, I. Alcohol behind Finland's high homicide rate. Science Nordic, October 2012. Retrieved from http://sciencenordic.com/alcohol-behind-finlands-high-homicide-rate.

Lifton, R. J. Thought Reform and the Psychology of Totalism. New York, NY: W. W. Norton & Company Inc., 1961.

Lombardo, M. V., Chakrabarti, B., Bullmore, E. T., Wheelwright, S. J., Sadek, S. A., Suckling, J., Baron-Cohen, S., MRC Aims Consortium. Shared neural circuits for mentalizing about the self and others. Journal of Cognitive Neuroscience 22(7):1623–1635, 2010.

Longabaugh, R., Wirtz, P. W., Zweben, A., Stout, R. L. Network support for drinking, Alcoholics Anonymous and long-term matching effects. Addiction 93(9): 1313–1333, 1998.

Lorenz, K. Analogy as a source of knowledge. Science 185:229–234, 1974.

Luhrman, T. M. When God Talks Back: Understanding the American Evangelical Relationship with God. New York, NY: Alfred A. Knopf, 2012.

Magura, S. Evaluating Alcoholics Anonymous's effect on drinking in project MATCH using cross-lagged regression panel analysis. Journal of Studies on Alcohol and Drugs 74:378–386, 2013.

Makela, K., Arminen, I., Bloomfield, K., Eisenbach-Stangl, I., Bergmark, K. I., Kurube, N., . . . Zielinski, A. (Eds.). Alcoholics Anonymous as a mutual-help movement: A study in eight societies. Madison, WI: The University of Wisconsin Press, 1996.

Markus, H., Crane, M., Bernstein, S., Siladi, M. Self-schemas and gender. Journal of Personality and Social Psychology 42(1):38–50, 1982.

Mausner, J. S., Kramer, S. Epidemiology: An Introductory Text. 2nd ed. Philadelphia, PA: W. B. Saunders Company, 1985.

McDowell, D., Galanter, M., Goldfarb, L., Lifshutz, H: Spirituality and the treatment of the dually diagnosed: an investigation of patient and staff attitudes. Journal of Addictive Diseases 15:55–68, 1996.

McGeoch, J. A. Studies in retroactive inhibition: I. The temporal course of the inhibitory effects of interpolated learning. Journal of General Psychology 9(1): 24–43, 1933.

McIntire, D. How well does A.A. work? An analysis of published A.A. surveys (1968–1996) and related analyses/comments. Alcoholism Treatment Quarterly 18: 1–18, 2000.

McKellar, J., Stewart, E., Humphreys, K. Alcoholics Anonymous involvement and positive alcohol-related outcomes: Cause, consequence, or just a correlate? A prospective 2-year study of 2,319 alcohol-dependent men. Journal of Consulting and Clinical Psychology 71:302–308, 2003.

McLellan, A. T., Lewis, D. C., O'Brien, C. P. Kleber, H. D. Drug dependence, a chronic medical illness: Implications for treatment, insurance, and outcomes evaluation. Journal of the American Medical Association 284:1689–1695, 2000.

Merrill, J., Fox, K., Chang, H. H. The cost of substance abuse to America's health care system: Medicaid hospital costs. Report 1. Center on Addiction and Substance Abuse at Columbia University, 1993.

Miller, W. R., Baca, J. C. Quantum Change: When Epiphanies and Sudden Insights Transform Ordinary Lives. New York, NY: The Guilford Press, 2001.

Moos, R. H., Moos, B. S. Participation in treatment and Alcoholics Anonymous: A 16-year follow-up of initially untreated individuals. Journal of Clinical Psychology 62:735–750, 2006.

Mowrer, O. H. The New Group Therapy. Oxford, England: D. Van Nostrand Co., 1964.

Moyers, W. C. Broken: My Story of Addiction and Redemption. New York, NY: Penguin Group 2007.

Najavits, L. M., Hien, D. Helping vulnerable populations: A comprehensive review of the treatment outcome literature on substance use disorder and PTSD. Journal of Clinical Psychology 69:433–479, 2013.

National Institute on Alcohol Abuse and Alcoholism. (2015). Alcohol Facts and Statistics, 2015. Retrieved April 13, 2015 from http://www.niaaa.nih.gov/alcohol-health/overview-alcohol-consumption/alcohol-facts-and-statistics.

National Institute on Alcohol Abuse and Alcoholism. What's "at risk" or "heavy" drinking? rethinking drinking: Alcohol and your health. Retrieved April 13, 2015 from http://rethinkingdrinking.niaaa.nih.gov/IsYourDrinkingPatternRisky/WhatsAtRiskOrHeavyDrinking.asp.

Narcotics Anonymous World Services. N.A. Groups and Medication [pamphlet]. Chatsworth, CA: N.A. World Services Inc., 2007.

Narcotics Anonymous World Services. Narcotics Anonymous, 6th Edition. Chatsworth, CA: Narcotics Anonymous World Services, 2008.

Narcotics Anonymous World Services. The Birth of Narcotics Anonymous in Words and Pictures. Chatsworth, CA: Narcotics Anonymous World Services, 1998.

Nowinski, J., Baker, S., Carroll, K. Twelve Step Facilitation Therapy Manual: A Clinical Research Guide for Therapists Treating Individuals with Alcohol Abuse and Dependence (Vol. 1). Rockville, MD: U.S. Department of Health and Human Services, 1992.

O'Brien, C. P. Perspective on addiction. In M. Galanter, H. D. Kleber, K. Brady (Eds) Substance Abuse Treatment. Washington, DC: American Psychiatric Publishing, 2015.

Ouimette, P. C., Moos, R. H., Finney J. W. Influence of outpatient treatment and 12-step group involvement on one-year substance abuse treatment outcomes. Journal of Studies on Alcohol 59:513–522, 1998.

Orange, A. The Orange Paper: One Man's Analysis of Alcoholics Anonymous and Substance Misuse Recovery, Programs, and Real Recovery. Accessed online at: http://www.orange-papers.org/. Last updated, 2014.

Pagano, M. E., Friend, K. B., Tonigan, J. S., Stout, R. L. Helping other alcoholics in Alcoholics Anonymous and drinking outcomes: findings from Project MATCH. Journal of Studies on Alcohol 65(6):766–773, 2004.

Pansera, C., La Guardia, J. The role of sincere amends and perceived partner responsiveness in forgiveness. Personal Relationships 19:696–711, 2012.

Pennartz, C., Ito, R., Verschure, P., Battaglia, F., Robbins, T. The hippocampal–striatal axis in learning, prediction and goal-directed behavior. Trends in Neuroscience 34(10):548–559, 2011.

Peterson, M. D., Vaughn, R. C. (Eds.). The Virginian Statute for Religious Freedom: Its Evolution and Consequences in American History. New York, NY: Cambridge University Press, 1988.

Piaget J., Kegan P. The Child's Conception of the World. London: Routledge, 1929.

Pilbeam, D. The Ascent of Man: An Introduction to Human Evolution. New York, NY: Macmillan, 1972.

Poser, E. G. The effect of therapists' training on group therapeutic outcome. Journal of Consulting Psychology 30(4):283–289, 1966.

Post, S. G. The ontological generality: Recovery in triadic community with a Higher Power, neighbor, and self. Alcoholism Treatment Quarterly 32:120–140, 2014.

Project MATCH Research Group. Matching alcoholism treatments to client heterogeneity: Project MATCH three-year drinking outcomes. Alcoholism, Clinical and Experimental Research 22:1300–1311, 1998.

Publicker, M., McCain, K., Potter, J. S., Forman, R., Vetter V., McNicholas, L., Blaine, J., Lynch, K. G., Fudala, P. Extended vs. short-term buprenorphine-naloxone for treatment of opioid addicted youth: A randomized trial. The Journal of the American Medical Association 300(17):2003–2011, 2008.

Putnam, R. Bowling Alone: The Collapse and Revival of American Community. New York, NY: Simon and Schuster, 2001.

Pype, K. Confession cum deliverance: In/Dividuality of the subject among Kinshasa's Born-Again Christians. Journal of Religion in Africa 41:280–310, 2011.

Quiroga, R. Q., Reddy, L., Kreiman, G., Koch, C., Fried, I. Invariant visual representation by single neurons in the human brain. Nature 435(7045):1102–1107, 2005.

Rambo, L. R., Bauman, S. C. Psychology of conversion and spiritual transformation. Pastoral Psychology, 61(5–6):879–894, 2012.

Rice, D. P. Economic Costs of Substance Abuse, 1995. Proceedings of the Association of American Physicians, 111(2):119–125, 1999.

Riessman, F. The "helper" therapy principle. Social Work 10(2):27–32, 1965.

Rizzolatti, G., Fabbri-Destro, M. Mirror neurons: From discovery to autism. Exp. Brain Res. 200:223–237, 2010.

Robertson, N. Getting Better: Inside Alcoholics Anonymous. Lincoln, NE: iUniverse.com, Inc, 2000.

Rode, D. The 12 steps as a path to enlightenment: How the Buddha works the steps. USA: createspace, 2012.

Rode, D. The Twelve Steps as a path to enlightenment. Retrieved from http://12steppath-toenlightenment.com/dorena.htm.

Ryberg, P. ASAM History, processed, 2001.

S., L. 12 Steps on Buddha's Path: Bill, Buddha, and We. Somerville, MA: Wisdom Publications, 2006.

Saitz, R. Alcohol screening and brief intervention in primary care: Absence of evidence for efficacy in people with dependence or very heavy drinking. Drug and Alcohol Review 29:631–640, 2010.

Schrad, M. L. Moscow's drinking problem. The New York Times, April 16, 2011.

Shinde, S., Andrew, G., Bangash, O., Cohen, A., Kirkwood, B., Patel, V. The impact of a lay counselor led collaborative care intervention for common mental disorders in public and private primary care: A qualitative evaluation nested in the MANAS trial in Goa, India. Soc Sci Med 88:48–55, 2013.

Sifton, E. The Serenity Prayer: Faith and Politics in Times of Peace and War. New York, NY: W. W. Norton & Company, 2003.

Silberstein, C., Metzger, E. J., Galanter, M. The greenhouse: A modified therapeutic community for homeless addicts. In G. De Leon (Ed.) Healing Communities: Therapeutic Communities for Special Populations in Special Settings. Westport, CT: Greenwood Publishing Group, 1996, pp. 263–272.

Silk, J. B. Making amends: Adaptive perspectives on conflict remediation in monkeys, apes, and humans. Human Nature 9:341–368, 1998.

Smart Recovery. 2014 Participant Survey. Retrieved from: http://www.smartrecovery.org/resources/participant-surveys.htm.

Smith, H. The Russians. New York, NY: Ballantine Books, 1984.

Solomon, M. AA: Not the Only Way. Fairbanks, AK: Capalo Press, 2005, pp. 39–41.

Spilka, B., Shaver, P., Kirkpatrick, L. A. A general attribution theory for the psychology of religion. Journal for the Scientific Study of Religion 24:1–20, 1985.

Spreng, R. N., Mar, R. A. I remember you: A role for memory in social cognition and the functional neuroanatomy of their interaction. Brain Research 1428: 43–50, 2012.

Stimpson, A., Kroese, B. S., MacMahon, P., Rose, N., Townson, J., Felce, D., Hood, K., Jahoda, A., Rose, J., Willner, P. (2013). The experiences of staff taking on the role of lay therapist in a group-based cognitive behavioural therapy anger management intervention for people with intellectual disabilities. Journal of Applied Research in Intellectual Disabilities 26(1):63–70, 2013.

Stinchfield, R., Owen, P. Hazelden's model of treatment and its outcome. Addictive Behaviors 23:669–683, 1998.

Stone, V. E., Gerrans, P. What's domain-specific about theory of mind. Social Neuroscience 1(3–4):309–319, 2006.

Stout, R. L., Braciszewski, J. M., Subbaraman, M. S., Kranzler, H. R., O'Malley, S. S., Falk, D. What happens when people discontinue taking medications?: Lessons from COMBINE. Addiction 109(12): 2044–2052, 2014.

Strupp, H. H., Hadley, S. W. Specific vs. nonspecific factors in psychotherapy: A controlled study of outcome. Archives of General Psychiatry 36(10): 1125–1136, 1979.

Subbaraman, M. S., Kaskutas, L. A. Social support and comfort in AA as mediators of "Making AA Easier" (MAAEZ), a 12-Step Facilitation intervention. Psychology of Addictive Behaviors 26(4):759–765, 2012.

Swora, M. G. Narrating community: The creation of social structure in Alcoholics Anonymous through the performance of autobiography. Narrative Inquiry 11(2):363–384, 2002.

Tamir, D. I., Mitchell, J. P. Disclosing information about the self is intrinsically rewarding. Proceedings of the National Academy of Sciences 109(21):8038–8043, 2012.

Taylor, S. M., Galanter, M., Dermatis, H., Spivak, N., Egelko, S. Dual diagnosis patients in the modified therapeutic community: Does a criminal history compromise adjustment to treatment? Journal of Addictive Diseases 16(3):32–38, 1997.

The Betty Ford Institute Consensus Panel. What is recovery?: A working definition from the Betty Ford Institute. Journal of Substance Abuse Treatment 33(3): 221–228, 2007.

Timko, C., Moos, R. H., Finney, J. W., Lesar, M. D. Long-term outcomes of alcohol use disorders: comparing untreated individuals with those in Alcoholics Anonymous and formal treatment. Journal of Studies on Alcohol, 61, 529–540, 2000.

Todd, E. The value of confession and forgiveness according to Jung. Journal of Religion and Health 24:39–48, 1985.

Tonigan, J. S. Benefits of Alcoholics Anonymous Attendance. Alcoholism Treatment Quarterly 19: 67–77, 2001.

Tonigan, J. S., Rice, S. L. Is it beneficial to have an Alcoholics Anonymous sponsor? Psychology of Addictive Behaviors 24(3):397–403, 2010.

Trimpey, J. The Small Book: A Revolutionary Alternative for Overcoming Drug and Alcohol Abuse. New York, NY: Dell Publishing, 1995.

Trivers, R. L. The evaluation of reciprocal altruism. The Quarterly Review of Biology 46: 35–37, 1971.

U.S. News. Top-ranked hospitals for psychiatry. U.S. News and World Health Report: Health. Accessed October 22, 2014 from http://health.usnews.com/best-hospitals/rankings/psychiatry.

Valliant, G. The Natural History of Alcoholism. Cambridge, MA: Harvard University, 1983.

Van Veen, V., Krug, M. K., Schooler, J. W., Carter, C. S. Neural activity predicts attitude change in cognitive dissonance. Nature Neuroscience 12(11):1469–1474, 2009.

Van Zee, A. The promotion and marketing of OxyContin: Commercial triumph, public health tragedy. American Journal of Public Health 99(2):221–227, 2009.

Vick, K. Opiates of the Iranian People, despair drives world's highest addiction rate. The Washington Post, September 23, 2005. Retrieved from http://www.washingtonpost.com/wp-dyn/content/article/2005/09/22/AR2005092202287.html.

Viola, J. J., Ferrari, J. R., Davis, M. I., Jason, L. A. Measuring in-group and out-group helping in communal living: Helping and substance abuse recovery. Journal of Groups in Addiction & Recovery 4(1–2):110–128, 2009.

Volkow, N. D., Fowler, J. S., Wang, G. J., Swanson, J. M., Telang, F. Dopamine in drug abuse and addiction: Results of imaging studies and treatment implications. Archives of Neurology 64(11):1575–1579, 2007.

Wang, S. H., Tse, D., Morris, R. G. Anterior cingulate cortex in schema assimilation and expression. Learning & Memory 19(8):315–318, 2012.

Weber, M. The Theory of Social and Economic Organization. New York, NY: Macmillan, 1947.

Weiss, R. D., Potter, J. S., Fiellin, D. A., Byrne, M., Connery, H. S., Dickinson, W., Gardin, J., . . . Ling, W. Adjunctive counseling during brief and extended buprenorphine-naloxone treatment for prescription opioid dependence: A 2-phase randomized controlled trial. Archives of General Psychiatry 68(12):1238–1246, 2011.

Whelan, P. J., Marshall, E. J., Ball, D. M., Humphreys, K. The role of AA sponsors: a pilot study. Alcohol and Alcoholism 44(4):416–422, 2009.

White, W. Slaying the Dragon: The History of Addiction Treatment and Recovery in America. Bloomington, IL: Chestnut Health Systems, 2014.

Wikler, A. Some implications of conditioning theory for problems of drug abuse. Behavioral Science 16:92–97, 1971.

Wilson, E. O. Sociobiology: The New Synthesis. Cambridge, MA: Belknap Press, 1975.

Woody, G. E., Poole, S. A., Subramaniam, G., Dugosh, K., Bogenschutz, M., Abbott, P., Publicker, M., . . . Fudala, P. Extended vs. short-term buprenorphine-naloxone for treatment of opioid addicted youth: A randomized trial. Journal of the American Medical Association 300(17):2003–2011, 2008.

Wurmser, L. The Hidden Dimension: Psychodynamics in Compulsive Drug Use. New York, NY: J. Aronson, 1978, republished 1995.

Zaki, J., Ochsner, K. N. The neuroscience of empathy: Progress, pitfalls and promise. Nature Neuroscience 15(5):675–680, 2006.

Zaridze, D., Brennan, P., Boreham, J., Boroda, A., Karpov, R., Lazarev, A., Konobeevskaya, I., . . . Peto, R. Alcohol and cause-specific mortality in Russia: A retrospective case-control study of 48 557 adult deaths. The Lancet 373:2201–2214, 2009.

INDEX

Piaget, Jean, 170
Placebo-controlled studies, 221, 222
Pledge (to renounce drinking), 129
Population genetics, 162
Positivism, 47, 136
Post, Stephen, 97
Post-traumatic stress disorder (PTSD), 46, 206
Prayer
  the brain and, 93, 172–76, 177, 178–83
  individual responses to, 178–83
  most commonly recited in AA, 93–94
  Step focusing on, 93–99
Prefrontal cortex, 24, 39
Primates, nonhuman, 159, 160, 163, 164, 167
Prohibition, 212
Project MATCH, 16, 185, 186
Protestantism, 86, 87, 202
Psychiatric perspective on addiction, 29–32
Psychoanalytic model of addiction, 23, 27–29
Psychological perspective on spirituality, 123–26
Psychotherapy, 222–24
  engagement in AA and, 67–69
  group, 60
  sponsorship compared with, 112
PTSD. See Post-traumatic stress disorder
Public health perspective on addiction, 23, 32–33
Putnam, Robert, 127

Qigong, 151
Quantum change, 79

Rambo, Lewis, 80
Randomized controlled trials (RCTs), 136, 184–85, 187
Rational Emotive Therapy, 212
Rational Recovery, 212–14
Reciprocal altruism, 162
Recovery. See also Abstinence/sobriety
  defining, 199–201
  in physicians, 44, 104, 139–40, 142–44
Recovery coaches, 154

Rehabilitation programs (rehabs), 103, 135, 148–55
  affiliation with academic medical centers, 150
  alternatives to, 153–55
  beginnings of, 148
  controversies over, 17–18, 150–51
  cost of, 153
  economic problems besetting, 152
  follow-up treatment in, 152
  luxury-oriented, 151, 152
  Minnesota Model in, 148–51
  positive aspects of, 151
Reinforcement, 53, 163. See also Conditioned responses
Relapse
  brain research on, 166, 176–78
  cognitive behavioral therapy on, 223
  in heroin addiction, 26–27
  psychoanalytic model on, 28–29
  in rehab patients, 152
  repeated, 195–96
Relief effect, 53
Religion, defined, 12. See also Spirituality
Research, 41–47, 103–4, 139–40
  approach to studying AA, 46–47
  economic support for, 144–45
  on effectiveness of AA, 185–88
  emphasis on biological factors, 158
  field studies, 42–44
  limitations of AA cooperation with, 41, 104, 136, 186, 201
  on medications, 145–46, 221, 222
  on the Minnesota Model, 151
  on NA, 45–46, 205–7
  on prayer effects on brain, 172–76, 178–83
  randomized controlled trials, 136, 184–85, 187
  on spirituality, 116–17, 122–23
  on sponsorship, 107
  on success rate of AA, 16–17
Restorative justice, 92
Retreats, 127, 129–30, 140, 211
Revia, 145, 221. See also Naltrexone
Riessman, Frank, 106
Rockefeller, John D., 4–5
Rourke, Mickey, 36
Rush, Benjamin, 29, 203

CPSIA information can be obtained
at www.ICGtesting.com
Printed in the USA
BVHW042118081021
618443BV00002B/2

9 780190 276560